Struck Down by the Gods

Causes and Prevention of Stroke

Professor Peter Gates

Peter Gates OAM, MBBS, FRACP, FAAN
Affiliate Professor of Neurology, Deakin University,
Waurn Ponds, Victoria, Australia,
Associate Professor of Neurology, Melbourne University,
Parkville, Victoria, Australia,

Address for correspondence:
PO Box 1224
Barwon Heads
Victoria, Australia 3227

Email: prof.petergates@gmail.com

Contents

Apoplexy

Apoplexy is the ancient term for stroke. It literally means Struck Down by the Gods.

Unlike heart attacks due to the disease of the hardening of our arteries (atherosclerosis). Stroke is damage to our brain resulting from either a blocked or a burst blood vessel.

Many diseases cause stroke, but one cause of stroke due to a blocked blood vessel is atherosclerosis or hardening of our arteries.

Atherosclerosis
The term atherosclerosis$_1$ is used frequently throughout this book. It refers to the increasing stiffness and hardness of the walls, and the subsequent accumulation of cholesterol in the walls of our arteries. This process can lead to progressive narrowing and in some case complete blockage of an artery.
Atherosclerosis is the main cause of heart attacks, angina and poor circulation to the legs. It is only one of the many causes of stroke.
The earliest changes of atherosclerosis are present in every single person by the age of 3 and increase in severity as we age.

In this book superscript[1] is used for the references, whilst subscript$_1$ refers to the footnotes

---

1   from the Greek words athere, meaning gruel or wax, and sclerosis, meaning hardening.

Copyright

This publication is copyright. Except as expressly provided in the Copyright Act 1968 and the Copyright Amendment (Digital Agenda) Act 2000, no part of this publication may be reproduced, stored in any retrieval system or transmitted by any means (including electronic, mechanical, microcopying, photocopying, recording or otherwise) without written permission from the author.

Every attempt has been made to trace and acknowledge copyright, but in some cases this may not have been possible. The Author apologizes for any accidental infringement and would welcome any information to redress the situation.

This publication has been carefully reviewed and checked to ensure that the content is as accurate and current as possible at the time of publication. We would recommend, however, that the reader verify any procedures, treatments, drug dosages or legal content described in this book. Neither the author, nor the publisher assume any liability for injury and/or damage to persons or property arising from any error in or omission from this publication.

Author: Peter Gates

Title: *Struck Down by the Gods – Causes and Prevention of Stroke*

ISBN 978-0-6455156-4-0 Paperback (black and white internal pages)

ISBN 978-0-6455156-5-7 Paperback (colour internal pages)

ISBN 978-0-6455156-6-4 eBook

BISG Codes:

MED000000 MEDICAL/General

MED056000 MEDICAL/ Neurology

Dewey Number: 610, 616

Foreword

We have known the author for more than 30 years and we have always respected his enormous contribution to education in stroke. He has already written a very successful book on general neurology and he is well known as a gifted teacher and communicator for both medical students and young neurologists. He is an independent thinker and does not shy away from communicating contrarian views. This certainly enlivens the book in a unique way and invites, in his own words, controversy. It is, therefore, a pleasure to be able to write a foreword to such a wonderful contribution.

The publication of this book "Struck Down by the Gods" lives up to its title. It is timely, as stroke is undergoing a revolution in knowledge and new treatments are transforming outcomes of this often-devastating condition. As well as treatment, the content spans "all one wants to know about stroke" from history, epidemiology, risk factors to stroke prevention. We particularly liked the organisation of the chapters to have contrarian thoughts and appendices with vignettes, particularly about the classical derivations of technical words and the history of concepts. We are sure that the author has been aware of the aphorism of Wilhelm von Humboldt that "only he or she who knows the past has a future." Indeed, there is a particularly strong emphasis on the historical development of concepts in stroke, which are embedded in each section. His contrarian thoughts are nicely highlighted within summary boxes, often insightful personal perspectives. There are extensive sections on lifestyle factors that contribute to stroke risk, particularly the problems with modern western "obesogenic diets." There are interesting discussions of epidemiological disparities in risk factors associated with stroke, such as differences in the levels of obesity, hypertension and hyperlipidaemia. He includes many interesting and littleΔknown facts such as the occurrence of stroke in domestic dogs.

Who should read this book? It is highly informative for the lay audience. However, based on our own enjoyment of the volume, we are sure that well-established neurologists will enjoy the journey. Even more importantly, it is a highly readable introduction to the topic for those just commencing their careers such as students of medicine and other healthcare disciplines as well as early career trainees. We unreservedly commend this book to these diverse audiences. Enjoyment is assured!

Geoffrey A Donnan AO FAHMS, Professor of Neurology, University of Melbourne
Stephen M Davis AO FAHMS, Professor of Translational Neuroscience, University of Melbourne and Director, Melbourne Brain Centre at Royal Melbourne Hospital
Richard Gerraty MD FRACP, Professor of Medicine, Monash University.

Acknowledgements

I wish to acknowledge the wonderful help from Sandy Coventry from Nitty Gritty Graphics[2], who is an amazing illustrator and also my close friend Kevin Sturges for his assistance with modifying images and IT support.

I need to thank Sophia Auld of Words Mean Business[3] for her amazing proof reading.

The project would not have been possible without access to the online resources of the University of Melbourne Library.

I would also like to acknowledge the support Sir Edward Byrne AC who has been a wonderful mentor, colleague, and close friend.

This book is dedicated to my long-suffering wife Rosie who has tolerated my long hours in my "den or man-cave" and who without her support it would not have been possible. It is also dedicated to my three wonderful children Bernard, Amelia, and Jeremy for still talking to me even after the many years I was not around during their early childhood.

2   https://nittygrittygraphics.com.au/
3   sophia@wordsmeanbusiness.com.au

Preface

My Journey in Stroke Research

I have been interested in stroke for over 40 years. In 1981, my mother passed away in her mid-50s from a severe stroke caused by a blockage in the major basilar artery in her brain. She had several health problems, including morbid obesity, high blood pressure, and diabetes, and she was a smoker. At that time, there was no treatment for her condition.

During my medical training, I worked with some of the best stroke specialists[4] and researchers. I was involved in important studies that helped doctors understand stroke better. These experiences deepened my interest in stroke research and led me to work on major clinical trials after returning to Australia.

Understanding Conflicting Opinions

There are many different opinions about stroke. Sometimes, doctors strongly disagree on the best treatment. For example, surgeons and physicians once argued about whether a surgery called carotid endarterectomy (removing plaque from an artery) was helpful. It took two major studies[1,2] to prove who would benefit from the operation.

This book is for people without a medical background. It explains the types of strokes, their causes, warning signs, and risk factors. However, it does not focus on treatment after a stroke has happened. All health care professionals involved in the care of stroke patients will benefit from this book.

A Journey of Discovery

Over many years of researching stroke (with a temporary focus on obesity, which increases stroke risk), I found a lot of surprising information. Some of it made me question what I had been taught.

I once read a quote that said:

> *"If researchers stopped doing new studies and just read what had already been written, they would make more discoveries."*

This book is the result of more than 12 years of research and over 40 years of experience treating stroke patients and participating in clinical trials.

---

4   H.J.M. "Barney" Barnett on the Extracranial to Intracranial (EC-IC) Bypass and NASCET studies and the team of Dave Sackett, Brian Haines, and Wayne Taylor from the department of clinical epidemiology and biostatistics at McMaster University, Hamilton, Ontario where I undertook a epidemiology course.

Contrarian Thoughts
Throughout the book, I include "contrarian thoughts" – ideas that challenge common beliefs in stroke medicine. My goal is to encourage scientific debate, not criticism.

Other quotations form the basis for the contrarian thoughts in this book.

"*The great tragedy of science, the slaying of a beautiful hypothesis by an ugly fact*"
... Sir Thomas Huxley 1825–1895

"*Discovery is seeing what everybody else has seen and thinking what nobody else has thought....*Albert Szent-Györgyi 1893–1986[5]

"*In today's environment, our talent for jumping to conclusions makes it all too easy to find false patterns in randomness. To ignore alternative explanations for a result or to accept 'reasonable' outcomes without question. That is, to ceaselessly lead ourselves astray without realizing it.*"
... Dr Regina Nuzzo from Gallaudet University, Washington.

---

5   Nobel Laureate 1937, the discoverer of vitamin C and the citric acid or Krebs cycle.

The Structure of the Book

The first three chapters explore the history of stroke medicine:

Ancient Times to the 14th Century – The "Age of Ignorance," when medical knowledge was very limited.

14th to 20th Century – The "Age of Enlightenment," when old ideas were questioned and medical science advanced.

20th and 21st Century – The modern era, when technology helped doctors see and treat the brain more effectively.

Next, the book explains how the brain and its blood vessels work. Other key chapters discuss:

- Two misleading studies
- The hardening of arteries and its link to stroke
- How to tell if something causes a stroke or is just associated with it
- How risk and benefits are measured in medical studies.

Later sections describe the different types of strokes, risk factors, early warning signs, and conditions that can be mistaken for a stroke. The final section focuses on how to prevent a first stroke and avoid a second one.

The Challenge of Misinformation

Before the internet, it was difficult to find all the research on a topic. Now, doctors can access thousands of studies instantly – but not all of them are accurate. This flood of information can be confusing, both for patients and doctors.

I hope this book helps answer common questions about stroke and how to prevent it. I have learnt many new things through this journey, and I believe this book will be useful to both stroke patients and their caregivers.

For those who want to dive deeper, extra information and my personal perspective on artery hardening and high blood pressure are available on my website[6].

No-One Lives Forever

Death is not the enemy. Human death is normal; we all die. The real enemies are premature death, disability, pain, human suffering, and the prolongation of dying. All the rest is mostly noise.

— George Lundberg. June 2023[7]

Understanding Death and Disease

Death is a natural part of life. Everyone dies eventually, but what we should try to prevent is dying too soon, living with pain, or suffering for a long time before death.

Most people will not stay perfectly healthy until the day they die. At some point, we will develop a serious illness. In 2019, 74% of deaths worldwide[8] were caused by chronic diseases – illnesses that do not spread from person to person. The leading causes of death globally are heart attacks, strokes, lung disease (mostly from smoking), and serious infections.

One of the goals of this book is to help people learn how to prevent strokes (and heart attacks), which can lead to early death and disability.

A person's risk of dying increases with age:[9,3]

- A 65-year-old has a **1 in 100** chance.
- An 85-year-old has a **1 in 10** chance.

While we cannot stop aging or change the genes we inherit, we **can** control how we live. Avoiding smoking and not gaining too much weight can help us live longer and stay healthier.

One of the best ways to live a long life, seen in all animals, is **eating fewer calories**. Eating less affects our genes and can actually slow down aging.[4] Throughout the entire animal kingdom, the secret to longevity is "caloric restriction" (eating less).

---

7   https://www.medscape.com/viewarticle/993639?form=fpf
8   https://www.who.int/news-room/fact-sheets/detail/the-top-10-causes-of-death
9   Based on UK Office of National Statistics data. It is likely to be similar in other 1st world countries.

This Book will be Criticised

Questioning Popular Beliefs

History shows that progress in medicine often begins with someone daring to question the status quo. When someone challenges common beliefs, they often face criticism. A good example is John Yudkin, who wrote a book about the dangers of sugar called Pure, White, and Deadly. Yudkin was pilloried by not only the food and beverage industry but also by Ancel Keys. If no one ever questioned old ideas, we might still believe in outdated medical practices. For example, the famous Greek physician, Galen misled the world of medicine for centuries until another scientist, Vesalius, proved him wrong. William Osler, a highly respected physician once believed morphine was the best treatment for diabetes, which we now know is completely false.

Even people who are not experts can question scientific studies. This book contains ideas that might go against mainstream views, especially about what causes hardened arteries (atherosclerosis) and high blood pressure. However, evidence shows that atherosclerosis starts decades before the onset of obesity, diabetes, smoking, high blood pressure and in the majority a high cholesterol.

In the world of nutrition, many studies look for links between habits and diseases, but just because two things are related does not mean one causes the other. Some researchers may disagree with what is written in this book, but they have to acknowledge the fact that association does not prove causation. If repeated studies find the same association, as was observed with smoking, causation is more likely. This book contains research undertaken by some of the greatest scientists and doctors over several centuries.

The Weight Loss Industry

The weight loss industry is worth billions of dollars. In the US, about 45 million people go on a diet every year, spending $33 billion on weight loss products. This industry – and even some researchers – may not like the simple truth: to lose weight, we need to eat less and exercise more. While the concept is simple, it is far from easy. We are surrounded by an obesogenic environment that makes unhealthy choices far too convenient,[10] making it harder to maintain a healthy weight.

Studies show that:
- 69% of Australians live within 1.5 km of a fast-food outlet.
- Canadian teenagers are more likely to eat fast food if it is less than 1 km from their home.

---

10 https://www.statista.com/statistics/1040896/australia-fast-food-outlet-accessibility-by-distance/

- People in Holland tend to have higher body weight if they live near multiple fast-food places.
- In the US, fast food is often closer to homes than sit-down restaurants or grocery stores.
- Food delivery apps make it easier to eat unhealthy meals without leaving the house or even the couch!

Imagine if millions of people adopted healthier habits – eating less, moving more, and maintaining a healthy weight. The food and pharmaceutical industries would lose billions in profits, and governments would save on healthcare costs. It's no surprise, then, that those with a financial interest in the status quo may try to discredit ideas that threaten their business model.

Keeping an Open Mind

The information within these pages is not mere opinion – it is based on centuries of medical research and clinical observation. I would encourage readers to approach this book with an open mind, focusing on the facts rather than clinging to outdated beliefs. This is what the author experienced during the many years of researching this book, I had to unlearn much of what I had been taught.

A famous poem tells the story of six blind men who each touched a different part of an elephant and argued about what it was like[11]. They were all partly right, but all were completely wrong. This reminds us to look at the bigger picture, with a willingness to look beyond our own perspective.

The ultimate goal of this book is to inspire positive change: to quit smoking, eat healthier, move more, and achieve a healthy weight. I speak from experience – I have lost and regained weight many times, but by committing to lasting lifestyle changes[12], I finally succeeded in keeping it off. Maintaining a healthy BMI[13] of 25 kg/m² or lower (or a waist circumference to height ratio of less than 0.5) can help us live longer, healthier lives with a reduced risk of heart attacks and strokes.

With such a massive undertaking, it is possible that some errors have slipped through. I hope that these will be forgiven and not used to discredit the entire work.

---

11 the 6 blind men of Indostan, the 1872 poem by John Godfrey Saxe.

12 I am a "chocoholic" and have struggled to maintain a healthy weight, at one point bordering on obese. I was motivated to lose weight by the evidence described in this book from World War II.

13 BMI or body mass index is one of several measures of obesity, (Kg/m2). It is calculated by dividing our weight in Kg by out height I metres multiplied by itself. E.g. a 1.7m tall person weight 90Kg has a BMI of 90/(1.7*1.7).

Stroke is not a Disease

A stroke is not a disease. It is a term used to describe what happens when the brain is damaged due to:

- A burst blood vessel that causes bleeding in the brain[14], or
- A blocked blood vessel[15] that stops blood and oxygen from reaching part of the brain.

About 80% of strokes happen because of blocked blood vessels, while 17% are caused by bleeding in the brain[5].

Many different diseases can lead to a stroke.

For strokes caused by blocked blood vessels:

- 25% are from a blood clot forming in the heart and embolising to the brain[16][6]
- 15% are from clogged large blood vessels leading to the brain.[7]
- 25% are from blockages in tiny blood vessels deep in the brain.[17]
- 30–40% have no clear cause.[18][8]

More details on stroke types can be found in Chapters 21 and 22.

---

14 The medical term is: haemorrhage.
15 The medical term is: infarction.
16 The medical term is: cardioembolic, cardio means heart and "embolos" meaning plug or obstruction.
17 The medical term is: lacunar infarction from the Latin word lacuna, which means "pit" or "hole".
18 from the Greek words kryptos, meaning "hidden", and genesis, meaning "origin".

ASCVD

ASCVD: What It Really Means

ASCVD (**A**therosclerotic **C**ardiovascular **D**isease) is a term often used when talking about strokes and heart attacks.

What is Atherosclerosis?

Atherosclerosis is the gradual damage to the blood vessels (arteries) as we age. This damage includes:

- Thickening and hardening of artery walls
- Cholesterol buildup under the artery lining[19]

Even though this book is mainly about stroke, atherosclerosis can affect the arteries to the heart, brain, and legs. Many people who have had a stroke may also have a heart attack, and vice versa.

Is ASCVD the Right Name?

A big issue with the term **ASCVD** is that doctors diagnose it only after symptoms appear. But the real disease – atherosclerosis – starts developing **decades before** symptoms show up.

This means most people have atherosclerosis without knowing it, and they **may never** have a stroke, heart attack, or circulation problems in the legs.

A better term might be **ASCVS (Atherosclerotic Cardiovascular Symptoms)** since it refers only to people who already have symptoms, not the actual disease.

This book will show just how early in life atherosclerosis starts – you may be surprised!

Blockage of blood vessels occurs when the inner lining[20] of our artery ruptures, triggering the formation of a blood clot that either blocks the artery where it forms, or it breaks off and travels downstream where it occludes the artery[21].

Blocked arteries to the brain cause stroke, blocked arteries to the heart cause angina, heart attack and sudden death.

Blocked arteries to the legs cause pain in the calves with walking that is relieved by rest, referred to as intermittent claudication, or they can result in gangrene of the toes and feet.

---

19 This subintimal cholesterol together with calcium, and cellular waste is referred to as a plaque.
20 called the intima or endothelium, it is a layer of specialised cells that allow the blood to flow smoothly in the arteries, it can be likened to Teflon. This subintimal cholesterol together with calcium, and cellular waste is referred to as a plaque.
21 This is referred to as embolism from the Greek word embolismos, which means "intercalation (essentially inserting)" or "interpressure".

Although symptoms are more common when the artery is very narrow, rupture of a plaque not causing severe narrowing – and undetectable with modern tests can precipitate symptoms.[9]

Contrarian Thought
There is a major problem with the term ASCVD We are diagnosed as having AtheroSclerotic CardioVascular Disease (ASCVD) when we first develop symptoms. This is the tip of the iceberg. Lurking below the surface is every one of us with the disease atherosclerosis affecting the arteries who have not yet, and may never experience a stroke, heart attack or poor circulation to the legs. **Thus, ASCVD is almost a misnomer**; it is not a disease. This book will reveal the disease, atherosclerosis commences decades before we develop the so-called risk factors currently believed to be the cause and decades before symptoms, you will be surprised just how early in life it does 1st develop.

Contrarian Thought
ASCVD is the label for those who have developed symptoms from the disease atherosclerosis. **Perhaps it should be renamed ASCVS, Atherosclerotic CardioVascular Symptoms.**

The Cart Cannot Come Before the Horse

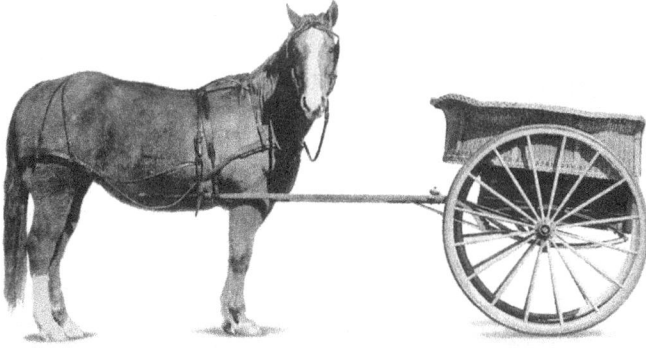

Understanding Atherosclerosis

A Simple Explanation:

Everything seems complicated until it is explained simply.

In **Section Four**, we will show clear evidence that atherosclerosis – the hardening and stiffening of arteries with cholesterol buildup – starts decades before symptoms appear and worsens with age.

- Over **90% of heart attacks** are caused by atherosclerosis.
- However, strokes can have many causes, and atherosclerosis is just one of them.

Atherosclerosis Starts Early in Life

The evidence is undeniable:

- Some people develop atherosclerosis **before birth**.
- **By age 3, early signs** are found in **everyone**.
- It worsens as we age and **may or may not** lead to heart attacks, angina, strokes, or poor circulation.

Do Risk Factors Really Cause Atherosclerosis?:

- Atherosclerosis develops **before** common risk factors like smoking, diabetes, high blood pressure and high cholesterol appear.
- Some people with **no risk factors** still develop atherosclerosis.
- This suggests that risk factors **do not cause** atherosclerosis but when these risk factors develop, they will worsen the atherosclerosis and increase the risk of developing symptoms.

What is the Real Cause?

One thing affects **100% of us** – the **physical stress on artery walls** from every heartbeat, starting before birth.

- **Turbulence** at artery branches also contributes to damage over time.

This Explains Many Medical Mysteries:

- **Heart attacks and strokes in healthy people** without risk factors such as high blood pressure or high cholesterol.
- **Heart attacks in young people** under 30 with no known risks.
- **"Unknown cause" (cryptogenic) strokes**, where it is likely that small plaques may rupture without being detected.
- **More strokes and heart attacks with increasing age**, as atherosclerosis worsens.
- **The "apparent" family history of heart disease and stroke**, despite little evidence of inherited genes directly causing it.

The vast majority of us **do not inherit genes** that cause atherosclerosis, although we may inherit genes that make us prone to more severe atherosclerosis because of the anatomy of the arteries to our heart and brain. More on that later.

Atherosclerosis is, in my opinion (see appendix A$_{22}$), the explanation for the cause of essential hypertension (high blood pressure). If we have essential hypertension, this is an indication that there is already stiffness of the walls of arteries.

Conclusion
The autopsy evidence is irrefutable, the logic is both sound and valid, the conclusion is inescapable: risk factors cannot be the primary cause of atherosclerosis, simply because the disease atherosclerosis commences decades before we develop these risk factors. This is not to say that they do not exacerbate atherosclerosis once they occur – they do.

---

22 The appendices are on the following website www.understandingneurology.com.au.

SECTION 1:
The History of Stroke

This section is for those who, like the author, enjoy reading about the history of medicine.

History has been arbitrarily divided into three eras: the Age of Ignorance, the Age of Enlightenment, and the Modern Era.

It is not necessary to read this section to benefit from reading the rest of the book.

1. The Age of Ignorance

Magic, Religion, and the Misunderstood Brain

In ancient times, people believed magic and religion played a big role in medicine. Civilizations like the Babylonians (1896–539 BCE), Egyptians (3100–322 BCE) and Greeks (700–480 BCE) thought diseases were caused by spirits and supernatural forces. Egyptian doctors and priests used spells and magic potions to drive away these spirits. It wasn't until the time of Hippocrates (460–370 BCE), known as the father of medicine, that people started thinking diseases had natural causes instead.

Some early ideas about the human body were very wrong. In ancient Greece, the philosopher Aristotle(384–322 BCE) believed that the heart controlled intelligence, while the brain was only there to cool the blood. The Egyptians thought the heart was the centre of emotions, memory, wisdom, and personality. They even believed that God spoke through the heart. Because of this, when Egyptians mummified a body, they left the heart inside, believing it would be judged in the afterlife. Meanwhile, they removed the brain by pulling it out through the nose and then threw it away, thinking it was useless!

The first known medical text to take a scientific approach instead of relying on magic was the Edwin Smith Surgical Papyrus. This ancient Egyptian text, bought (or possibly stolen) by Edwin Smith in 1862, was written around 1700 BCE. It contains one of the earliest references to the brain. One case describes a person with a head wound where doctors touched the brain, causing the patient to shake violently – most likely having a seizure.

The Greek doctor Herophilus (335–280 BCE), known as the father of anatomy, was one of the first to dissect human bodies. He correctly identified the brain as the organ responsible for intelligence. Egyptians also knew that the heart, pulse, and blood circulation were important and that the heart and blood vessels were connected.

Hippocrates was likely one of the first people to describe the symptoms of a stroke. He called it "apoplexy," meaning to be "struck down." Back then, people believed strokes were punishments from the gods. Hippocrates also noticed that strokes sometimes had warning signs, now called transient ischemic attacks (TIAs). He understood how serious strokes were, saying mild ones were hard to treat and severe ones were impossible to cure. Even today, strokes remain a major health issue, though modern medicine has made great advances in treatment and prevention.

References to strokes can also be found in even older texts. A Babylonian record from 605 BCE describes Menanu, king of Elam who had a stroke, lost his ability to speak, and later died. The Bible also contains a passage,[23] written around 600 BCE, that could describe a stroke. It mentions a person whose right hand withered and whose tongue stuck to the roof of their mouth – probably a stroke affecting the left side of the brain.[10]

Throughout history, people have often believed whatever famous doctors and scientists said, even when they were wrong. For example, Hippocrates thought veins carried air because they appeared empty in dead animals. One of the most influential (but often incorrect) doctors was Galen of Pergamon (131–201 A.D.). His ideas about "humors" (blood, phlegm, yellow bile, and black bile) controlling health and disease were accepted for centuries. The church supported Galen's ideas because they fitted with religious teachings. Questioning Galen's theories was considered heresy, which could lead to execution.

Galen believed that strokes were caused by too much phlegm blocking the arteries in the brain. However, he never actually saw a brain haemorrhage because ancient Greeks rarely dissected human bodies. Instead, Galen studied the wounds of injured gladiators and based much of his work on animal dissections, leading to many mistakes in his understanding of the human body.

Galen's ideas were finally challenged in the 14th century by Andreas Vesalius (1514–1564) and in the 17th century by William Harvey (1578–1657). Vesalius studied human anatomy by dissecting cadavers (dead bodies), sometimes taken from graveyards or hospitals. He drew detailed images of the body, creating the first accurate medical anatomy textbook. Harvey later proved that the heart pumps blood through the body, an idea that was rejected at first. Some of his patients even left him because they refused to believe him. Michel Servetus (1511–1553), who described the circulation to the lungs, was sentenced to be burnt at the stake for his views by Protestant reformer John Calvin.[11]

Surgery in the Age of Ignorance

Brain surgery has been performed for thousands of years. A 7,000-year-old skull[24] found in France shows evidence of two surgeries where pieces of bone were removed[25]. The person survived at least one of these procedures. Many ancient civilisations, including the Incas and Sumerians, performed similar surgeries, often in an attempt to release evil spirits.

Before modern anaesthesia, surgery was incredibly painful. Ancient people used alcohol and opium to make patients drowsy, but they were still awake during surgery. They were held down by strong men while the surgeon worked, often screaming in pain. The discovery of anaesthesia in the 18th century finally made surgery bearable, leading to huge advances in medical treatment.

---

23 Psalm 126: 1 Samuel 25: 37–38.
24 Found in Ensisheim, in the French region of Alsace and dating back to Neolithic times.
25 Removing bone from the skull is called trepanation, from the Greek word trypanon, which means "to bore" or "to auger".

Medicine has come a long way from the days of magic and superstition, but history shows how long false ideas can last – especially when powerful people support them. Even today, it's important to question information and rely on science to find the truth.

STRUCK DOWN BY THE GODS

2. The Age of Enlightenment

The Facts and Theories of Science

Pioneering Spanish histologist and neuroscientist Santiago Ramon y Cajal once said, "The facts remain and theories pass away." This means that in science, facts stay true, but theories can change over time. Francis Darwin, son of Charles Darwin, also pointed out that the person who gets credit in science is not always the one who has an idea first, but the one who convinces others about it[26].

Medical Discoveries

The Age of Enlightenment was a time when people started questioning old medical beliefs, especially those of Galen, which had dominated for over 1,300 years. This period, also called the Medical Renaissance, led to major discoveries about how the human body works. Important inventions such as the microscope and printing press helped create and spread new medical knowledge.

There is some debate over who created the first microscope in the late 1500s. It may have been Hans Lippershey (1570–1619) or the Janssen father-and-son duo, Hans (1601–1645) and Zacharias (1585–1638). The printing press, invented by Johannes Gutenberg (1400–1468) in 1440, allowed knowledge to spread quickly. Despite these advancements, medical treatments were still primitive. For example, when King Charles II had a stroke in the 1600s, doctors treated him with bloodletting, laxatives, and a potion made from a bezoar stone (a hardened mass found in an animal's stomach) that they mistakenly believed could cure poison.

Understanding the Brain

Ancient scientist Galen knew the brain controlled thinking, movement, and emotions but did not know that different parts of the brain had different functions. Before the 1700s, many believed the whole brain worked as one. Franz Joseph Gall (1758–1828) and Johann Spurzheim (1776–1832) in Vienna, Austria, challenged this idea by suggesting that specific parts of the brain controlled specific functions. They developed phrenology – the false idea that a person's skull shape could reveal personality traits. Although phrenology was incorrect, it helped scientists realise that different parts of the brain serve different purposes.

Jean-Baptiste Bouillaud (1796–1881) suggested in 1825 that the left side of the brain controlled speech and movement on the right side of the body.[12] Paul Broca (1824–1880) confirmed this in 1861[13] and received most of the credit. The term

---

26 This was in response to allegations that Sir Charles Darwin had plagiarised the work of Alfred Russel Wallace (1823–1913) and Patrick Matthew (1790–1874).

"Broca's aphasia" is still used today to describe speech problems caused by damage to the left frontal lobe of the brain. Broca was a surgeon at Paris's Bicétre Hospital, which had previously been the prison where the Marquis de Sade was incarcerated. It is most famous as the first lunatic asylum to treat patients with psychiatric illnesses humanely, a policy pioneered by its superintendent, Philippe Pinel.

Discovering Blood Circulation

William Harvey[27], (1578–1657) an English doctor, accurately described how blood circulates through the body in the 1600s. He discovered that arteries carry blood away from the heart while veins bring it back. However, he did not understand how oxygen entered the blood through the lungs. Earlier scientists – like Arab physician Ibn al-Nafis (1210–1288), Italian surgeon Realdo Colombo (1516–1559)[28],[14] and the Spaniard Michel Servetus (1509–1533) – had suggested this, but their ideas were not widely known at the time.

The complete understanding of circulation came in the 1600s with the discovery of tiny blood vessels called capillaries by Italian physician and biologist Marcello Malpighi of Bologna (1628–1694). Capillaries connect arteries and veins, allowing blood to flow throughout the body.

Many scientists contributed to our knowledge of the brain's blood vessels. In 1664, English physician Thomas Willis (1621–1675) described the "Circle of Willis," a ring of arteries supplying blood to the brain[15] (Figure 5.3, Chapter 5). Another physician, Johann Wepfer (1620–1695) of Schaffhausen, Switzerland, had described the same structure six years earlier[29],[16] but did not make a drawing, so, Willis received more credit. Wepfer was also the first to classify strokes into two types: those caused by blocked blood flow and those caused by bleeding in the brain.[17]

The "father" of modern anatomical pathology[30],[18] is Giovanni Battista Morgagni, who was the first Professor of Anatomy at Padua University in Italy (1682–1771)[18] He studied the brains of more than 700 patients.[19],[20] Morgagni carefully noted the symptoms of his patients' illnesses and then attempted to identify what had caused their diseases at autopsy.[31]

---

27 Harvey was the physician to kings James 1 and Charles 1.
28 Colombo first coined the term 'circulation' (Khan, I. A., et al. (2005). "Evolution of the theory of circulation." *Int J Cardiol* 98(3): 519–521).
29 Published in: On the Seats and Causes of Diseases Investigated by Anatomists.
30 The study of organs and tissues to work out the causes and effects of particular diseases.
31 In 1761 he published his book of pathology, *De Sedibus et Causis Morborum per Anatomen Indagatis* "On the Seats and Causes of Diseases Investigated by Anatomists".

The History of Anaesthesia

Before anaesthesia[32], surgery was extremely painful. For centuries, people experimented with painkillers, but none worked well enough for surgery. Operations like tooth removal, gallstone removal, or amputations were done while patients suffered extreme pain. Ancient texts mention substances like hemp or cannabis, while the Romans used mandragora (from mandrake plants) mixed with wine to numb pain. Later, people used opium from poppies. Homer mentioned nepenthe that was probably hemp or cannabis.

The first possible anaesthetic was discovered by English chemist Sir Humphry Davy (1778–1829)[33] in 1799 when he inhaled nitrous oxide, a gas thought to be poisonous.[21] He realised it made him laugh uncontrollably and numbed his limbs, so he called it "Laughing Gas." Davy believed it could relieve pain during surgery, but no one in medicine took him seriously. Instead, people used it for entertainment.

Meanwhile, a failed medical student named "Professor" Gardner Quincy Colton (1814–1898) toured the US demonstrating laughing gas. In 1844, a dentist named Horace Wells (1815–1848) saw one of Colton's shows and noticed that a man under the gas didn't feel pain from his bruises. The next day, Wells had his own wisdom tooth removed painlessly using laughing gas given to him by "Professor Colton". This was likely the first time an effective anaesthetic was used.

However, when Wells tried to demonstrate it publicly, the patient woke up in pain. Wells was booed from the auditorium with shouts of "Humbug!" On October 16, 1846, Wells' partner William Morton (1819–1869) successfully used ether[34] as an anaesthetic while the surgeon Dr. John Collins Warren painlessly removed a tumour from a patient's neck. This took place at Massachusetts General Hospital in Boston in a room now called the "Ether Dome."

Interestingly, both nitrous oxide and ether had been noticed by English scientists decades earlier but were ignored. It took American dentists and a charlatan to rediscover them and change medicine forever.

The Discovery of X-Rays

One of the most important medical discoveries was x-rays. In 1895, German physicist Wilhelm Röntgen (1845–1923)[22] found that invisible rays could pass through solid objects. He took the first x-ray; it was of his wife's hand. This discovery changed medicine by allowing doctors to see inside the body without surgery.

---

32 The loss of feeling or awareness caused by drugs.
33 Davy is better known for inventing a miner's safety lamp in 1815.
34 Ether had originally been suggested by Faraday in England as early as 1818.

Shortly after, French physicist Henri Becquerel (1852–1908) discovered radioactivity in 1896. [23] He worked with Pierre (1859–1906) and Marie (1867–1934) Curie[35], who discovered radium and polonium, which were later used in cancer treatments. Sadly, Marie Curie died from exposure to radiation, unaware of its dangers.

Conclusion

Over the centuries, medicine has learnt a great deal from autopsies. In the 21st century very few patients undergo an autopsy. Blood tests, CT scans, and MRI scans enable many diagnoses to be made before death. These tests are done on corpses as part of the modern post-mortem.[24]

---

35 Both Polish-born French physicists.

3. The Modern Era

This chapter describes the incredible changes in stroke treatment from the late 20th to the early 21st century. In the past, stroke patients had little hope – some recovered, others died, and many were left disabled. However, major breakthroughs during this time transformed stroke care.

One of the biggest advances was the ability to take detailed images of the brain and blood vessels. Scanners like CT (computerised tomography), MRI (magnetic resonance imaging)[36], ultrasound, and PET (positron emission tomography) became widely used in the second half of the 20th century. These tools allowed doctors to see what was happening inside the brain, leading to better treatments. New drugs were developed to dissolve blood clots, and later, doctors learned how to physically remove them using a procedure called mechanical thrombectomy. Hospitals created specialised stroke units with teams of doctors, nurses, and therapists. In some places, stroke treatment even started in ambulances, speeding up care and improving survival rates.[25]

The Discovery of CT Scanning

One of the most important medical breakthroughs was the CT scan, which allowed doctors to see inside a living brain for the first time. Before this, they had to rely on symptoms to guess whether a stroke was caused by a blocked or burst blood vessel. CT scans use X-ray beams from different angles to create a 3D image of the brain.

Godfrey Hounsfield[37], an engineer who had worked in radar and computers, invented the CT scan while working for EMI, the company famous for recording The Beatles.[26,27] The first scanners were called EMI scanners. In 1972, Dr Jamie Ambrose, the radiologist from the Atkinson Morley Hospital, London, presented the images of a brain tumour inside a post-mortem brain to the Annual Congress of the British Institute of Radiology in London and the Radiological Society of North America in Chicago. In Chicago, he received a rare accolade at scientific meetings – a standing ovation.

It was not long before hospitals in London[38], Manchester[39], Glasgow[40], Boston[41], and Minnesota[42] ordered CT scanners. Before CT scans, doctors had to perform painful and risky procedures, like injecting dye into the arteries to see blood vessels[43]

---

36 MRI was originally called NMRI (nuclear magnetic resonance imaging), but "nuclear" was dropped to avoid negative associations.
37 1919–2004.
38 Atkinson Morley.
39 Manchester Royal Infirmary.
40 Institute of Neurological Sciences (INS) at the Southern General Hospital.
41 Massachusetts General Hospital
42 Mayo Clinic, Rochester.
43 Cerebral angiography.

or injecting air into the fluid around the brain[44]. These dangerous tests were soon abandoned in favour of CT scans.

In 1977, the author was in the room at St Vincent's Hospital[45] when the first CT scan of a brain was shown; the looks on the senior doctors' faces were unforgettable.

The Development of Ultrasound

Ultrasound, which uses sound waves to create images, became another important tool for detecting stroke. It helps doctors find blockages in the arteries leading to the brain and can also check for problems in the heart. The idea of ultrasound goes back to the 18th century when an Italian monk, Lazzaro Spallanzani, studied bats and discovered they could navigate using sound. Almost 150 years later, Donald Griffin at Harvard University established that bats emit sound waves at a frequency that is too high for people to hear.[28,29]

Modern ultrasound technology was developed in Austria by the Dussik brothers. One was a physicist and the other was a doctor.[30] Over time, ultrasound became a common and safe way to examine patients without using radiation. A more detailed account was published by Paul Newman and Grace Rozycki from Atlanta, Georgia.[31]

MRI and Its Impact

Magnetic resonance imaging (MRI) revolutionised stroke treatment by providing even clearer images than CT scans. It works by using strong magnets to align tiny particles in the body, then using radio waves to create detailed images. MRI is especially useful for detecting small strokes and for distinguishing old from new strokes when a CT scan cannot. A special MRI technique can detect brain cells that can recover after a stroke if blood flow is restored[46].

MRI was inspired by the work of Nikola Tesla[47], who developed the rotating magnet concept. In fact, the strength of MRI machines is measured in "Tesla" units. While MRI is extremely useful, it is not available in all hospitals or countries due to its high cost.

MRI scanners in most hospitals are 1.5–3.0 Tesla. There are research MRI scanners as high as 10.5 Tesla, with a 14 Tesla MRI under construction in Radboud University, Nijmegen, the Netherlands.[48]

---

44 Pneumoencephalography (PEG) was done by inserting a needle in the low back; a lumbar puncture.

45 Fitzroy, Victoria, Australia.

46 This is called the ischaemic (lack of blood flow) penumbra, from Latin paene 'almost' and umbra 'shadow'.

47 It is said the idea of using an alternating current to power the rotating magnet came to him whilst he was walking in a park in Budapest and reciting 'Faust', written by Johann Goethe. Elon Musk named his car Tesla after Nikola Tesla, a Serbian-American inventor and electrical engineer who discovered the rotating magnetic field, among many other amazing discoveries

48 https://healthcare-in-europe.com/en/news/14-tesla-mri-strongest-scanner.html#:~:text=In%20the%20 DYNAMIC%20project%2C%20researchers,field%20strength%20of%2014%20Tesla.

PET Scans

Positron emission tomography (PET) involves injecting a tiny, safe amount of a radioactive substance into the body to create images. While PET scans can show blood flow and brain activity, they are mostly used for research rather than routine stroke treatment. They have been more useful in detecting cancer but could play a bigger role in stroke care in the future.

Clot-Busting Drugs

In the 18th century, scientists noticed that blood did not clot immediately after death, [20] but it wasn't until the 20th century that doctors began experimenting with clot-dissolving drugs.[32] Streptokinase, found in bacteria, was the first such drug, discovered in the 1930s.[32] In 1958, Alan Johnson and Ross McCarty from Bellevue Hospital in New York conducted a remarkable study.[33] They caused blood clots to form in the veins of volunteers and then injected streptokinase into a different vein to see if it would dissolve the clots. Their experiment proved that the drug worked. However, a study like this would not be allowed today because it would not meet ethical standards. Later, another drug called urokinase was found in soybeans.[34] Early attempts at using it to dissolve blood clots failed.[35,36]

In 1995[49], a study showed that a drug called tissue plasminogen activator (t-PA) could dissolve blood clots in stroke patients, marking the first effective stroke treatment.[37] The excitement was huge, but not everyone agreed with the findings.[38,39] Some experts questioned the study's methods, leading to further reviews.[40–43] These confirmed that thrombolysis (clot-busting treatment) reduces death and disability if given quickly after a stroke. Thrombolysis was rapidly introduced in the treatment of acute stroke. Unfortunately, it tends to work best in patients with less severe stroke.

Clot Removal (Thrombectomy)

Thrombectomy, or clot removal/retrieval, is a procedure where doctors insert a thin tube into the arteries to physically remove a blood clot from the artery to the brain. Dr Y. Pierre Gobin, born in France but working at the University of California Los Angeles (UCLA), was pivotal in the development of clot retrieval[50].[44]

The first attempts in the 1990s were unsuccessful, but by 2001, Dr. Gobin had designed a tool like a tiny corkscrew to grab and pull out clots. The first successful procedure in 2001 instantly restored movement in a paralysed patient.

At first, studies on thrombectomy gave mixed results,[45–47] but by 2015, five major studies[48–52] confirmed its benefits. Although it is not suitable for all stroke

---

49 The author was at the 1995 International Stroke Conference in San Antonia, Texas, when the results of the study were first announced. Many neurologists wore badges indicating the dose they would need based on their weight; surprisingly there were many very overweight neurologists.
50 The story is told in detail on the UCLA neuroradiology website.

patients, it has become a major treatment to reduce both the severity of, and the risk of dying from, a stroke.

The Internet and Medical Advancements

The development of the Internet and the World Wide Web [51] has also played a role in stroke treatment. Instant access to medical information[52] helps doctors stay updated on new research and treatments. However, the internet also contains a lot of misinformation, making it important to rely on trustworthy sources.

Conclusion

The past few decades have seen incredible progress in stroke treatment. Advances in imaging, medication, and surgery have saved countless lives and reduced disability. From a time when stroke patients had little hope, medicine has now reached a point where many strokes can be treated effectively, especially if help is sought quickly. Unfortunately, not all strokes respond to these amazing treatments, and the emphasis must remain on prevention.

---

51 In the 1900s, Nikola Tesla theorised a "world wireless system." Guglielmo Marconi beat Tesla when he sent the Morse-code signal for the letter "S" from England to Canada via a radio transmission in 1901. The concept of the world wide web was first enunciated in 1945 by Vannevar Bush, an American engineer. ARPANET, an experimental computer network was created by the Advanced Research Projects Agency (ARPA) in the 1960s and used by the US Department of Defence. In the 1970s, engineers Robert Kahn and Vinton Cerf at Stanford University created the Transmission Control Protocol (TCP) and the Internet Protocol (IP) which is how data is sent between networks. In 1989 the computer scientist Tim Berners-Lee working at CERN ("Conseil Européen pour la Recherche Nucléaire", or European Council for Nuclear Research), the European Particle Physics Laboratory created the world wide web as we know it today.
52 In fact, too much information.

SECTION 2:
The Brain and Blood Vessels

This section describes the structure of our brains and our blood vessels.

4. The Brain

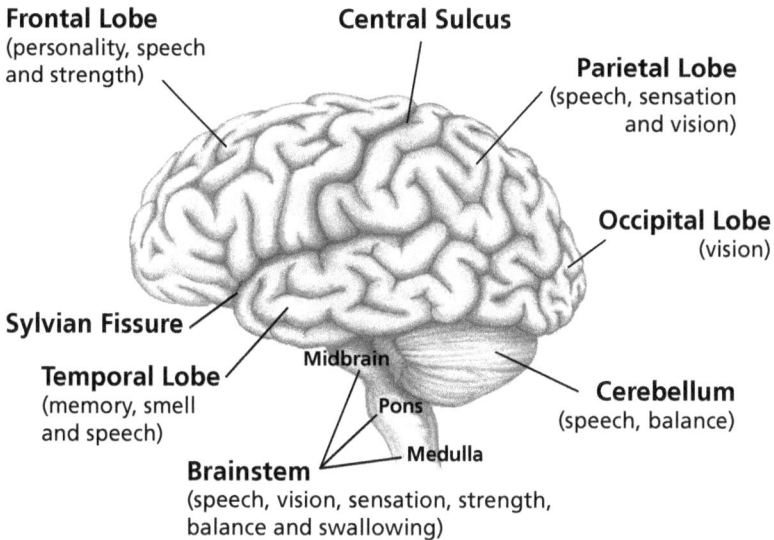

Figure 4.1: The brain viewed from the left-hand side. Source: Gates, P., *Clinical Neurology. A Primer*, 2010, p. 97.[53] It shows the major parts of the brain and the functions that they control.

The brain controls everything we do, from moving and speaking to remembering things and feeling emotions. Understanding how the brain works helps us understand the many different symptoms that can occur with a stroke.

Structure of the Brain

The brain (Figure 4.1) looks like a cauliflower and feels soft and jelly-like. It has different parts that control different body functions:

- **Brainstem** – This is like the "stalk" of the cauliflower. It connects the brain to the spinal cord. All messages travel to and fro through the spinal cord from the head and body to the brain.
- **Cerebral hemispheres** – These are the two large "bunches" on top of the brainstem. They control opposite sides of the body. The left side of the brain controls the right side of the body, and the right side of the brain controls the left side of the body.
- **Cerebellar hemispheres** – These are two smaller "bunches" at the back of the brainstem. They help with balance, coordination, and speech.

A stroke in different parts of the brain causes different problems. If a stroke affects the left cerebral hemisphere, the right side of the body may be weak or completely paralysed. If it affects the cerebellum, a person may experience clumsy movement.

Four Lobes of the Brain and Their Functions

The two cerebral hemispheres are divided into four main lobes, each responsible for different functions (Figure 4.1):

- **Frontal lobe** – Controls movement, speech, emotions, and personality.
- **Parietal lobe** – Controls speech and sensation (touch, pain, and temperature).
- **Occipital lobe** – Controls vision.
- **Temporal lobe** – Controls speech, memory, hearing, and smell.

The side used for production of speech is called the dominant hemisphere. Most people use the left side of their brain for speech. Scientists don't know why! People with a dominant left brain tend to be logical and organised, while those with a dominant right brain are often creative or artistic.[54]

When certain brain areas are damaged by a stroke, speech may become slurred (as if we are drunk), a condition called **dysarthria**.

Brain Pathways

The brain sends and receives messages through pathways that run down to the fingers and toes. There are three main pathways:

1. One sends signals from the **frontal lobe** to move muscles on the opposite side of the body.
2. The other two carry messages about sensations like pain, temperature, and body position back to the brain.

These pathways pass through the brainstem, which also controls eye and facial movements, balance, hearing, and sensation in the head, face and mouth.

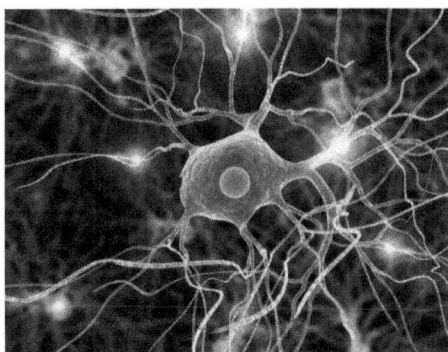

Figure 4.2 A neuron or brain cell showing the cell body with lots of tentacles called axons and dendrites.

Brain Cells

The brain and spinal cord are made up of billions[55] of tiny cells called **neurons** and **glial cells**. Neurons send messages using electrical signals. They look like tiny octopuses, with a central body and many "tentacles" called **axons** and **dendrites**.

- **Axons** send messages to other neurons. Some are up to one meter long!
- **Dendrites** receive messages from other neurons.

Glial cells support and protect neurons. Some even clean up dead neurons. The brain is protected inside the skull, and the spinal cord inside the backbone. Together, they form the **central nervous system**, which controls everything the body does. A stroke can damage both neurons and glial cells, affecting brain function. Rarely, the spinal cord can be damaged by either a blocked or burst blood vessel.

5. The Blood Vessels of the Body and Brain

The Circulatory System

This chapter explains how blood flows through the body, which is called the circulation or circulatory system. You can think of the circulation like an irrigation system. The **heart** is the pump, **blood vessels** are the pipes, **blood** is the fluid moving through them, and the **cells** are the fields that need nutrients. The circulatory system not only delivers oxygen and nutrients but also removes carbon dioxide and waste products away from the cells. Blood returns to the heart through veins, where it is sent to the lungs to get rid of carbon dioxide before picking up fresh oxygen.

Arteries, Veins, and Capillaries

Arteries carry blood **away** from the heart, while veins bring it **back**. The pulmonary[53] artery takes blood to the lungs to pick up oxygen, and the pulmonary veins return it to the heart. From there, the oxygen-rich blood is pumped through the **aorta,** the body's largest artery, to the rest of the body, including the brain.

Arteries branch into smaller and smaller vessels, eventually becoming **capillaries** – tiny blood vessels so narrow that blood cells must line up single file to pass through. Capillaries allow oxygen and nutrients to reach the cells while picking up carbon dioxide and waste. After this exchange, capillaries join together to form **veins**, which carry blood back to the heart. Very small arteries are called **arterioles**[54]. These arterioles play an important role in controlling the pressure in the arteries[55].[56]

The pressure in **arteries** is high, which is why blood **spurts** when an artery is cut. The pressure in **veins** is much lower, so blood **seeps** out more slowly when they are cut. Arterial blood is bright red because it carries oxygen, while venous blood is darker since it contains less oxygen.

Amazing Facts

If we stretched out all the blood vessels in the body, they would be about **60,000 miles (96,561 km) long** – more than twice the distance around the Earth! Every day, the heart pumps about **1,800 gallons** (6,814 litres) of blood, and over a lifetime, it moves roughly **43 million gallons** (162,772,707 litres). Just like old pipes, the blood vessels can wear out over time.

---

53 From Latin pulmonarius, from pulmo, pulmon – 'lung'.

54 From Modern Latin arteriola, diminutive of arteria – "an artery" – or from French artériole, diminutive of artère.

55 The muscular and elastic layers in arterioles contract when the pressure of blood in the arteriole increases and relax when the pressure falls, this is the Bayliss response. This is an important protective mechanism to prevent the transmission of blood under high pressure to the smaller, more fragile vessels downstream, the capillaries.

The Heart: The Body's Pump

Understanding how the heart works can help us understand strokes. Sometimes, blood clots form in the heart and travel through the arteries to the brain, causing a stroke.

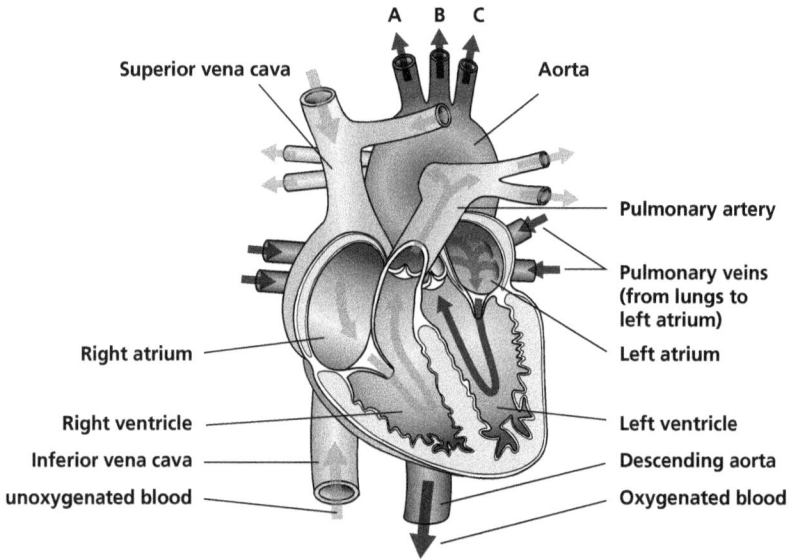

Figure 5.1 An illustration of the heart showing its chambers and major blood vessels. Illustration Sandra Coventry.

The heart has **four chambers** (Figure 5.1): two smaller upper chambers called **atria** and two larger lower chambers called **ventricles**. Blood low in oxygen enters the **right atrium** via very large veins called the superior and inferior vena cava. The blood in the right atrium is pumped via the **right ventricle** to the lungs through the **pulmonary artery.** In the lungs, blood picks up oxygen and releases carbon dioxide. The oxygen-rich blood then returns to the **left atrium** and is then pumped via the **left ventricle** to the entire body. The left ventricle's wall is thicker because it has to pump blood farther and at a much higher pressure. One-way valves in the heart keep blood flowing in the right direction.

Blood: The Body's Transport System

Blood is made up of **plasma** (a liquid that transports a small amount of oxygen, proteins, nutrients etc.) and three types of cells:
- **Red blood cells** carry most of the oxygen attached to a protein called **haemoglobin**.
- **White blood cells** help fight infections.
- **Platelets** help blood clot when we get a cut.

The total number of cells in the entire body is 30–35 trillion and nearly 70% of those are red blood cells.

Blood clots stem bleeding, but if they form inside arteries, they can block blood flow to the brain, causing a stroke (or heart attack when they block the artery to the heart).

Blood Vessels: The Body's Pipes

Arteries

Arteries have thick, strong walls with muscle and elastic layers to handle high pressure. They are lined with **endothelial cells**, which can be likened to Teflon because they allow blood to flow smoothly along the length of the artery. Smoking and high blood pressure can damage these cells, leading to **atherosclerosis**, a condition where arteries become stiffer and clogged with cholesterol.

The **aorta** is the body's largest artery. It comes up from the left ventricle, forms an arch,[56] and then curves downward, sending blood throughout the body (Figure 5.2).

Blood reaches the brain

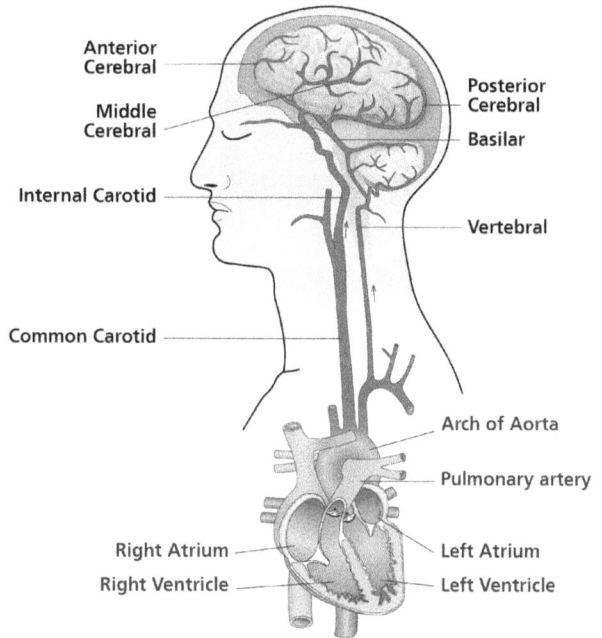

Figure 5.2 An illustration of the major blood vessels arising from the heart and going up the left side of the neck to the brain. The veins are not shown. Illustration Sandra Coventry.

through four main arteries – two **carotid arteries** in the front of the neck and two **vertebral arteries** in the back of the neck (Figure 5.2).

The carotid arteries in the front of the neck divide into two major arteries: the external carotid that supplies the face, scalp, and neck and the internal carotid that supplies most of the brain on the same side via the anterior and middle cerebral arteries. The two vertebral arteries at the back of the neck join together inside the

---

56 This is called the arch of the aorta and it bears the brunt of the high pressure as blood is forcefully pumped out of the left side of the heart. It is thus not surprising that this part of the aorta is a common site to see severe damage to its wall (atherosclerosis).

skull to make the basilar artery, from which the posterior cerebral artery arises. The anterior, middle and posterior cerebral arteries form a loop called the Circle of Willis, which supplies blood to different areas of the brain (Figures 5.3–5.5).

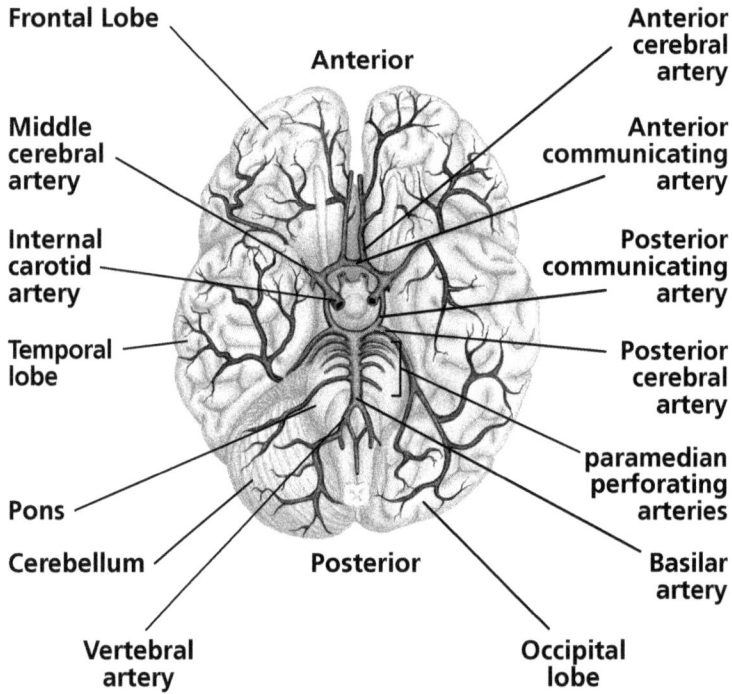

Figure 5.3 The Circle of Willis on the under surface of the brain.
Illustration Sandra Coventry.

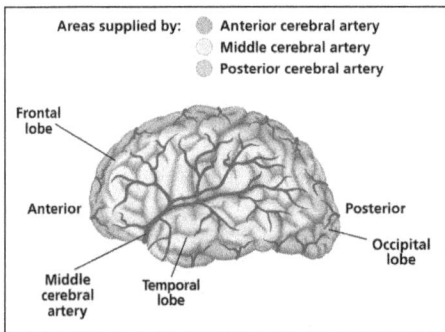

Figure 5.4 The brain and its blood supply from the lateral (outside) view.
Illustration Sandra Coventry.

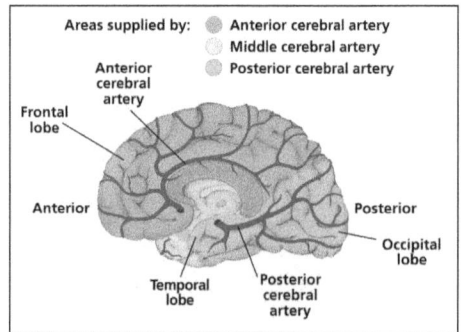

Figure 5.5 The brain and its blood supply from the medial (inside) of the brain.
Illustration Sandra Coventry.

Veins: The Return Path

Veins have thinner walls and carry blood under low pressure[57] back to the heart. The **superior vena cava** brings blood from the upper body, while the **inferior vena cava** brings blood from the lower body. Even though venous blood has less oxygen, it still has the same sugar and cholesterol levels as arterial blood. Interestingly, arteries develop **atherosclerosis**, but veins do not – more on that later.

The **cerebral veins** drain blood from the brain into large vessels called **venous sinuses**, which eventually return the blood to the heart through the **jugular veins** and superior vena cava.

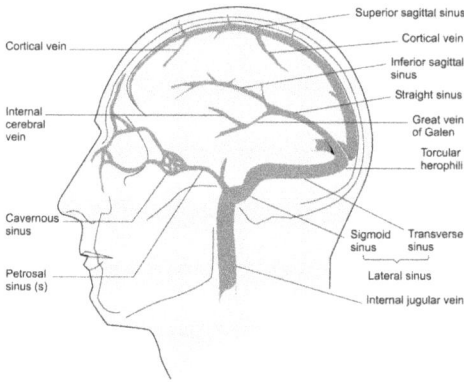

Figure 5.6 The veins that drain blood from the brain.

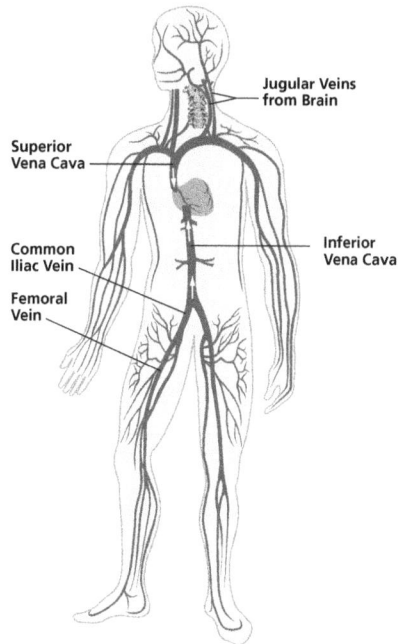

Figure 5.5 The veins of the body. Illustration Sandra Coventry.

The Body's Cells: The Final Destination

The body has about **37.2 trillion cells**, and about **60% of the body is water**. Cells need a steady supply of oxygen and nutrients, and constant removal of carbon dioxide and waste. Some cells – like those in the gut – live only a few days, while brain and heart cells can last a lifetime.[57]

There is a third set of vessels that have nothing to do with stroke or heart attack. These tiny vessels that drain fluid from around the cells, sit outside the arteries and veins. In the body they are called lymphatics[58] and in the brain they are called glymphatics.[58]

---

57 The pressure in the veins (8–10mmHg) is much lower than that in arteries (120–140mmHg).

58 From the Latin word lymphaticus, meaning "connected to water." The lymphatic system is part of the immune system that helps protect us from infection and cancer. The lymphatics drain into lymph nodes (also called glands), which enlarge with infection or cancer.

SECTION 3:
Two Misleading Studies and The Northern Tribes of Kenya and Inuit

---

Contrarian Thought
We would probably not have the dietary guidelines we have today if: • Ancel Keys' flawed Seven Countries Study had not been published, • Keys had studied the Inuits, the tribes of Tanzania and northern Kenya, or • More researchers had read Lieutenant Colonel Nikolai Anitschkow's 1933 *mea culpa* on the role of dietary cholesterol in atherosclerosis.

In his 1921 book The Friendly Arctic, the Arctic explorer Vilhjalmur Stefansson opined:

"There is no field of human thought
in which sentiment and prejudice
take the place of sound judgement and
logical thinking so completely as in dietetics."

This section discusses Anitschkow's rabbit experiment and Keys' flawed Seven Countries Study. Appendix A provides detailed information explaining how I reached the conclusion that these studies are misleading. I am not alone in questioning their validity.[59-61]

This section also examines societies where diets are high in cholesterol and saturated fat, yet the incidence of heart attacks and strokes remains low.

6. Rabbits, Cholesterol and a Russian Colonel

In 1913, Lieutenant-Colonel Nikolai N. Anichkov (Nikolay Anitschkow in the German literature) from the Imperial Military Medical Academy in St Petersburg published a study on the effect of feeding (overdosing) cholesterol to rabbits.[62] This chapter is derived from the English translation.[63]

Anitschkow's experiment has been described as one of the major medical discoveries of all time.[64] The Anitschkow and Chalatow paper stated: "After only four to eight weeks of feeding cholesterin (the ancient word for cholesterol) dissolved in oil[59] we produced in the experimental animals a rich infiltration...with liquid spherical crystals...in the aortic walls. The rabbits were fed egg yoke[60] in addition to their usual vegetable diet ad libitum[61],". It was known that egg yoke contained large amounts of cholesterol. The cholesterol levels needed to produce these changes were huge[62]. Much higher than what we consume in our everyday lives.[65]

In 1933, Anitschkow published a follow-up paper admitting that ageing alone could cause artery hardening in rabbits[63], even without high cholesterol diets[64].[66] This important detail was mostly overlooked.

On the basis of this study, we have been told we should limit the cholesterol in our diet. In the chapter on cholesterol, we will discuss how little the cholesterol in most of our diets influences the level of cholesterol in our blood.

---

59 Food that rabbits would not normally eat.
60 The old way of spelling yolk.
61 As often as necessary or desired.
62 16–18mmol/L (619–696mg/dL).
63 The verbatim quote from this 1933 paper can be found in appendix A.
64 Page 307 in the chapter titled Experimental arteriosclerosis in animals.

7. An American Physiologist, Saturated Fat and the Seven Countries Study

Ancel Keys and His Impact on Nutrition

Ancel Keys was a determined and influential scientist. Born in Colorado Springs, US, in 1904, he lived to be 100 and was still working at 97! He was a physiologist[65] at the University of Minnesota, where he studied nutrition and how diet affects health.

Keys became well known for his Minnesota Starvation Experiment and the K-rations he created for soldiers. In 1940, the US Army asked him to design a lightweight, nutritious food for paratroopers. The Quartermaster's Subsistence Laboratory named them "K-rations" after him, and Wrigley's Chewing Gum Company packaged them. However, they tasted terrible and were discontinued after the war.

Keys wrote an important book, *The Biology of Human Starvation*,[67] based on experiments beneath the football stadium at the University of Minnesota where 36 volunteers[66] reduced their food intake to mimic the struggles of Europeans during World War II. The men in the study lost a lot of weight and looked extremely thin by the end.

The Mediterranean Diet and BMI

Keys was one of the first to promote the Mediterranean diet, which he also followed. He spent 20 years convincing scientists to use Body Mass Index (BMI) as a measure of obesity. Today, however, waist-to-hip ratio is considered more useful because it measures fat around the organs. Interestingly, his own studies did not show a clear link between obesity and heart disease! [61]

Keys also spent years opposing a major health campaign in the US that linked weight control to preventing heart disease.[61] Despite his efforts, today we know that weight management plays an important role in heart health.

Controversy Over Fat and Heart Disease

Before conducting proper research, Keys had already decided that eating too much saturated fat increased the risk of heart attacks. In 1953, he published his study[68] suggesting that fat consumption was linked to heart disease, but his data

---

65 A physiologist studies functions and processes in living things.
66 Conscientious objectors.

came from unreliable sources[67]. A detailed analysis of the 22 countries originally included in Keys' Seven Countries Study concluded that there was no link between dietary fat and death from atherosclerotic heart disease.[59]

Keys was part of the Nutrition Advisory Committee of the American Heart Association (AHA). In 1957, the AHA recommended eating less fat – not because they were convinced fat caused heart attacks[68], but because it was higher in calories than protein or carbohydrates, and consuming too many calories leads to obesity[69].[69,70]

Looking back, it's likely that Keys' famous Seven Countries Study would not be published today because of its flawed research methods. In a 1986 paper, [71] Keys even admitted that his study showed an *association* between fat and heart disease but did not *prove* that fat caused heart disease. We'll explore the difference between association and causation in Chapter 19.

If Keys had studied groups like the French (who eat lots of fat but have low heart disease rates, known as the "French Paradox"), the Inuit, and certain African tribes who eat a lot of cholesterol and saturated fat but have low rates of atherosclerosis, his conclusions might have been very different. This is discussed in the next three chapters.

To this day, the dietary guidelines[72] still advise against consuming saturated fat. As Yerushalmy and Hilleboe[59] pointed out in 1957:

"But quotation and reputation of the suggestive association soon create the impression that the relationship is truly valid and ultimately it acquires status as a supporting link in the chain of presumed proof."

In other words, repeated suggestions that one thing is linked to another lead people to believe it is true. This supposed link can then become part of a chain of assumptions in future research.

Let's hope the views of Keys do not prevail as long as those of Galen.

The Role of Sugar

Many scientists believed that fat and cholesterol caused clogged arteries because they are found in atherosclerosis. However, avoiding smoking and obesity is far more important for preventing heart disease (Chapters 30 and 33).

Keys' influence led to the removal of fat (and salt) from many foods. To keep food tasty, manufacturers replaced them with sugar and artificial sweeteners, creating new health problems. Researchers like John Yudkin[73] and Gary Taubes[74,75] warned that sugar was harmful. Yudkin's book was titled *Pure, White and Deadly*[73]. They were both criticised – especially by Ancel Keys and the food industry, who stated that sugar is a natural substance, so it cannot be deadly.

---

67 Non-vital statistics from unidentified sources and the figures on fat consumption from the 1949 Nutrition Division, Food and Agriculture Organization of the United Nations report.

68 In fact, the report said that there was no proof that excess saturated fat was the cause of heart attacks.

69 The exact wording in the report can be found in Appendix A.

While sugar is a natural substance, the problem is the huge amounts people consume. Sugar has more than 60 different names and is often hidden in processed foods. In the 18th century, people in the UK ate about 1kg of sugar per year. Today, that number is around 70kg! The same trend has happened in the US over the last 100 years.[76] We will explore the impact of sugar on obesity in Chapter 30.

Contrarian Thought
It seems that because fat and cholesterol are in the atheroma of arteries, research has been directed to prove that fat and cholesterol in the diet are the cause!
This is not to say we should not try and reduce cholesterol.
The best way to reduce the risk of atheroma building up on the inside of arteries is to avoid smoking and obesity. More on this later.

I've always wondered why fat, even though it tastes great, is bad. In fact, it is not bad, if like everything we do not overindulge. Taking fat (and salt) out of food removes two things that influence taste. The others are sugar, sour, and umami (the savoury flavour we get from monosodium glutamate). This has caused major problems. To make up for the lost flavour, the food industry started adding sugar and artificial sweeteners instead.

8. The Inuit and the Tribes of Tanzania and Northern Kenya

The Samburu, Rendille and Turkana Tribes

The Samburu, Rendille and Turkana tribes in northern Kenya eat a diet high in saturated fat and cholesterol. Even so, heart attacks and strokes are rare when they live traditionally.

The Samburu mainly eat meat, milk, and blood from cattle. Blood is mostly protein. Both the Samburu and Turkana have normal cholesterol levels between ages 15 and 70, and around 15% of people live past 60. The Rendille have slightly higher cholesterol levels in their 50s, but they drop later. These levels are similar to those of people on low-fat diets.

Despite eating a lot of fat and meat, members of these tribes weigh between 40–57 kg. Their blood pressure stays low and doesn't increase with age, unlike in Western societies.[77–80] A 1929 study of over 1,000 people living near Lake Victoria found no high blood pressure, heart disease, or stroke. In their early sixties, the average blood pressure was 106/67 compared to the much higher average blood pressure of 140/90 in Europeans of a similar age.[81]

A 1965 study of 600 Maasai[70] people found almost no heart disease,[82] low cholesterol levels, and little high blood pressure,[83] even though they ate a lot of animal fat – up to 300 g of saturated fat and 600mg of cholesterol per day![84] Autopsies of 50 Maasai who died from accidents or illness showed their hearts were smaller, and their arteries were mostly healthy compared to that of Westerners, simply because they did not have high blood pressure.[85]

When comparing the Maasai to rural and urban Bantu people (Table 8.1), the Maasai had the lowest rates of obesity and high blood pressure. This is despite their high-fat diet based on the traditional staple foods of milk, dairy products and meat from their animals, with a high fat content. The rural Bantu ate low-fat, high-carbohydrate diets, while urban Bantu ate both high fat, and high carbohydrate diets, and they had the highest rates of obesity and high blood pressure.

As shown in Table 8.1, when the Maasai and Bantu moved to cities, became less active, and ate more food (in particular carbohydrate), their blood pressure, obesity and cholesterol levels increased. This proves their excellent health wasn't due to "good genes" but rather their traditional lifestyle and stable weight[86,87].

---

70 Also spelt Masai.

	Diet	Energy expenditure (calories/day)	Obese (%)	High blood pressure (%)
Masai	High fat/ low carbohydrate	2,565	3	4
Rural Bantu	Low fat/high carbohydrate	1,500	12	16
Urban Bantu	High fat/high carbohydrate	891	34	21

Table 8.1 Comparison of diet, energy expenditure, obesity, and high blood pressure in the Maasai and Bantu.[83]

The Inuit

The Inuit[71] traditionally ate Arctic char (fish), seal, polar bear, and caribou – mostly raw. A 1958 study found their diet was high in protein, moderate to high in fat, low in carbohydrates and had very few calories.[88] Caribou and polar bear meat is lean, but seal blubber is high in fat. Their estimated daily intake was 250 g of protein, 125g of fat, and 54g of carbohydrates – around 1,300 calories. Because they ate so little and were highly active, they remained thin, with an average weight of 68kg.[89]

The Inuit of Alaska[90] and Greenland[91] had[72] low rates of heart disease. Some believed this was due to their high intake of omega-3 fats, but omega-3 supplements later failed to prevent heart attacks.[92–94]

The Inuit had very low cholesterol and blood pressure, even though they ate foods high in cholesterol. In a study of 2,500 Inuit, their average blood pressure was between 110–124/71–78 mmHg. Obesity was rare, with less than 5% of men and 21% of women being overweight by modern standards. In 1963, the median BMI of Inuit in Greenland was 23.7 kg/m² for men and 23.1 kg/m² for women.[95]

Autopsies of Inuit who died in accidents or from violence showed very little artery disease.[96] Although some believed their genes helped them handle high-fat diets, a 1928 study disproved this. Two Arctic explorers, Vilhjalmur Stefansson and Rudolph Anderson, only meat and fat[73] for a year under medical supervision in the metabolism ward of the Russell Sage Institute of Pathology in Bellevue Hospital, New York. They remained healthy, active, and did not develop diabetes

---

71 Eskimo is a blanket term used to refer to Indigenous people living in the Arctic and Polar regions of the world. Inuit is a term used to refer to original inhabitants of Canada and Greenland. The term Eskimo is regarded by some as a derogatory term. Inuit is both singular and plural.

72 Note the word "had" – once the Inuit adopted a western lifestyle, they developed severe atherosclerosis and suffered heart attacks and strokes.

73 They consumed 2,000–3,100 calories per day: 15–25% from protein, 75–85% from fat, and only 1–2% from carbohydrate.

or high blood pressure.[97] Stefansson had already lived for nine years on a pure meat and water diet while exploring the Arctic.[98]

When Inuit moved to cities and ate processed foods, their obesity rates increased.[99] In 1855, the Inuit of Greenland consumed only 6g of sugar per day. By the 1970s, this had jumped to 164–175g (40–44 teaspoons), along with more processed carbohydrates. This led to an increase in heart disease.[100]

The Inuit obtained glucose (carbohydrates) from raw meat, which contains glucose stored as glycogen. Cooking meat destroys glycogen, turning it into lactate instead.

9. The French Paradox

The French Paradox refers to the low rates of heart disease in France, despite their high intake of cholesterol and saturated fats[101] – the very foods that American dietary guidelines warn against. Strangely, this has never led to questioning of those guidelines.

Unlike what is often recommended for heart health, the French eat little fruit or fibre. A 2003 study[102] by Paul Rozin in Philadelphia and French colleagues found that the French eat smaller portions in restaurants, buy less food from supermarkets, and have smaller serving sizes in cookbooks. They also eat more slowly, though they probably haven't heard of Horace Fletcher, who famously promoted chewing each bite 100 times![103] Some people think red wine might explain the paradox – a theory the wine industry loves.[101,104,105]

The real explanation is simple. The French eat fewer calories and are thinner. In 2003, only 7.4% of French adults were obese, compared to 22.3% in the US. However, as the French have started eating more – over 3,500 calories per day – obesity has, like a soufflé, been rising rapidly. By 2020, obesity had increased to 10%, with 40% of the population overweight.[74]

Once again, a so-called healthy eating theory is disproven by real-life facts. A high-fat diet was not linked to higher heart disease risk after all!

---

74 OECD Health Policies and Data https://www.oecd.org/en/data/indicators/overweight-or-obese-population.html.

10. Hara Hachi Bu

The Okinawan Way of Life and Longevity

Okinawa is a group of 160 tropical islands in the southernmost part of Japan. The people of Okinawa follow a tradition called **"Hara hachi bu"**, a Confucian saying they repeat before every meal. It reminds them to stop eating when they are **80% full** – the opposite of the "empty plate" habit, where people feel they must finish all their food!

Before World War II, Okinawans had the **highest life expectancy** in Japan and five times more people living to 100 years old than anywhere else in the country.[106] This wasn't due to genetics. In fact, Okinawans were **very poor**, and their traditional diet was **low in calories**.

Okinawan schoolchildren ate only **62% of the calories** that other Japanese children ate, while adults consumed **83% of Japan's average calorie intake**. The Body Mass Index (BMI) of adult Okinawans remained a lean **21 kg/m²** throughout life.[107] Their diet included pork, seaweed (mozuku), seafood, tofu, vegetables, and small amounts of grains, salt, and sugar.

However, things changed when the US occupied Okinawa from the end of World War II until 1972. Many Okinawans started eating more and adopted an **American-style diet**. By 1998, life expectancy in Okinawa had **dropped to the same as the rest of Japan**, and obesity levels had increased. This was linked to a more Westernised diet.[108]

Other Long-Living People

Many other cultures have long life expectancies. In the 16th century, an Italian nobleman Luigi Cornaro[75] wrote one of the first diet books, *La Vita Sobra* (*The Sober Life*). At 35, he improved his poor health and reportedly lived to **102** by eating just 342 g of food and drinking 400 ml of wine daily. At that time, most people only lived to 50–60 years, rarely reaching 70–80 years[76].

Another example is Emma Morano[77], who was the world's oldest living person before she passed away in 2017 at age **117**. Born in 1899, she followed the same diet for 90 years – three eggs a day (two raw, one cooked), fresh pasta, and raw meat. Despite this unusual diet, she remained thin, weighing **50 kg** at **1.73 m tall** (BMI **16.7**).

The Tsimané people of the Bolivian Amazon also live long, healthy lives. They rely on foraging and farming, and obesity, high blood pressure, and diabetes

---

75 https://www.lovefood.com/gallerylist/84379/horrible-historic-diets-youre-glad-you-never-had-to-try.
76 https://localhistories.org/a-history-of-life-expectancy/#:~:text=However%2C%20historians%20think%20it%20was,people%20born%20died%20in%20childhood.
77 Ms. Morano died 15th April 2017 age 117 years and 137 days!

are rare. Their cholesterol levels are low, and their hearts stay healthy, with 80-year-olds having the arteries of a 50-year-old American![109]

Other places with many centenarians include Silanus in Sardinia, Loma Linda in California, (the vegetarian Seventh-day Adventists),[110] and parts of Costa Rica.[111] While genetics may play a role, all these groups share one key factor – they stay thin.

Contrarian Thought
The study of these different cultures suggests that   **staying slim is the key to living a long, healthy life** – no matter what type of food you eat.

SECTION 4:
Hardening of our Arteries

"A man is as old as his arteries." – Thomas Sydenham (1624–1689)

One of the major causes of stroke is the blockage of blood vessels affected by atherosclerosis.

The terms *arteriosclerosis* and *atherosclerosis* have often been used interchangeably, leading to confusion. In this book, *atherosclerosis* and *hardening of the arteries* are used synonymously.

This entire section is dedicated to the hardening of our arteries. It will reveal many facts that reflect the famous quotation of Sir Thomas Huxley (1825–1895):

"The great tragedy of science – the slaying of a beautiful hypothesis by an ugly fact."

Once you understand and accept that the main cause of atherosclerosis is progressive damage to our artery walls – resulting from repeated physical pounding of the arterial walls with each heartbeat – everything falls into place.

This process begins while we are still in the womb, worsens with age, and is present to varying degrees in 100% of people. It explains:

- Why children have strokes.
- Why strokes and heart attacks occur in seemingly healthy individuals without any of the so-called risk factors.
- The likely reason why people have cryptogenic (unknown cause) strokes, and
- Why only a handful of genes have been identified in a small number of patients with rare causes of stroke – despite an apparent link between stroke and family history.

STRUCK DOWN BY THE GODS

11. Hardening of our Arteries – Ugly Facts

What You Should Know

Hardening of the arteries, also called **arteriosclerosis** or **atherosclerosis**, is a major cause of **strokes and heart attacks**. It happens when the arteries become stiff and **cholesterol builds up in their walls.** This makes the arteries narrower and can even cause them to become completely blocked over time. This section of the book will explore what causes it and challenge some common beliefs.

Many people think hardening of the arteries is a disease caused by old age, family history, obesity, high blood pressure, diabetes, high cholesterol, lack of exercise, and smoking. But the truth is it's more complicated than that.

Famous writer Aldous Huxley[78] once said that science often faces **"ugly facts"** that challenge what we think we know. Below are some surprising facts about hardening of the arteries that don't always fit with the usual explanations. More details can be found in Appendix G.

Surprising Facts About Hardening of the Arteries

- The **first signs** of hardening of the arteries appear **decades before** high blood pressure, obesity, diabetes, or smoking.
- **Healthy people** with none of the usual risk factors can still develop atherosclerosis, have heart attacks, or suffer strokes. A significant number of patients with a stroke under the age of 55 do not have risk factors. In the 18–24, 25–34, and 35–44 year age groups, the percentage of patients without risk factors was 27%, 24% and 14%, respectively.[112] Up to 25% of people who have a heart attack[113] have no known risk factors.
- Atherosclerosis can exist **without any symptoms**. Extensive subclinical (asymptomatic) atherosclerosis is present in 58% of 40–59-year-olds considered at low risk (as assessed by both the Framingham Heart Study and European 10-year risk scores).
- 17.6% of patients admitted to hospital with coronary artery disease had a low LDL cholesterol of <70 mg/dL (3.9 mmol/L).[114]
- It is **not just a modern disease** – it has been found in ancient mummies.
- It is **not unique to humans**—it also happens in animals.
- It is **not caused by eating cholesterol, meat, or fat**. For example, the Inuit people and the Northern Kenyan tribes eat mostly meat and fat but have very low rates of heart disease and stroke.

---

78 Born 1894, died 1963.

- Almost everyone has some degree of hardened arteries, but only **some people** develop serious symptoms.
- Hardening of the arteries **does not happen evenly** – some areas get worse than others, even though all parts of the artery are exposed to the same blood.
- **Veins do not develop atherosclerosis**, except in rare cases, even though they carry the same blood as arteries.
- Some arteries, like the internal mammary artery (behind the breastbone), the radial artery (in the forearm), and the pulmonary artery that delivers blood from the heart to the lungs, rarely develop atherosclerosis unless exposed to **high pressure**.
- It **doesn't only affect older people** – it can start also **before birth** and is seen in **children as young as three**! (Chapter 14)
- **Major weight loss** (like during World War II, (Chapter 17) can **reverse** atherosclerosis. Even weight loss, as occurs with bariatric surgery[116–118] can **stop it from getting worse**.[119]
- Cholesterol-lowering drugs can reduce heart attacks and strokes, but they **only slightly reverse** atherosclerosis in most patients.[120]

12. What is Hardening of Arteries?

This chapter explains how **hardening of the arteries** happens as we age. It occurs when the artery walls become stiff, and **cholesterol builds up**, beneath the inner lining of the artery, the intima, narrowing the arteries.

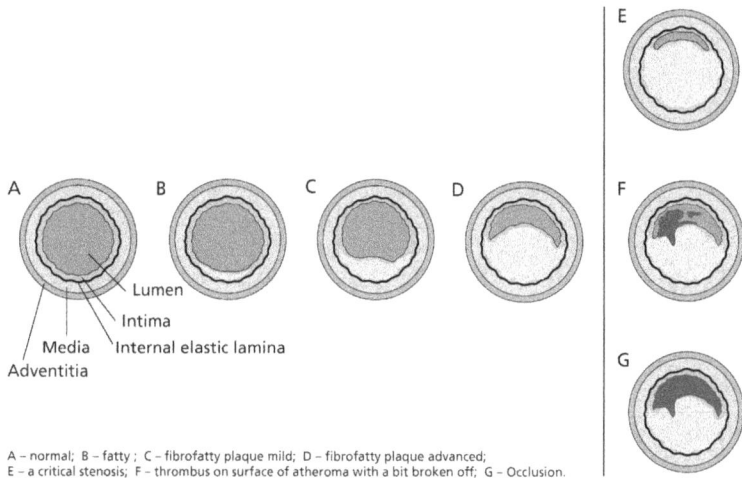

A – normal; B – fatty ; C – fibrofatty plaque mild; D – fibrofatty plaque advanced; E – a critical stenosis; F – thrombus on surface of atheroma with a bit broken off; G – Occlusion.

Figure 12.1: A normal artery (A) and the progressive development of atherosclerosis from fatty streaks (B) to severe atheroma (E) almost blocking the lumen, then rupture of the fatty plaque and thrombus (blood clot) formation (F), resulting in complete blockage (G).

A Normal Artery

Figure 12.1A shows a **normal artery**. The inside of an artery is called the **lumen**, where blood flows. The artery walls have **three layers**:

1. **Intima (inner layer)** – A thin, smooth layer of special cells (endothelial cells). It can be likened to Teflon because it allows blood to flow easily, but it thickens with age.[121]
2. **Media (middle layer)** – Contains muscle cells and stretchy fibres (collagen and elastin) that help arteries expand and contract with each heartbeat.
3. **Adventitia (outer layer)** – A tough, fibrous layer that gives structure and support.

In **young people**, arteries are straight, flexible, and elastic. Artery walls stiffen as we age, making it harder for them to expand and contract. This leads to **higher blood pressure** inside the artery and in the long-term further damage to the walls (Chapter 16).

Arteriosclerosis vs Atherosclerosis

The terms **arteriosclerosis**[79] and **atherosclerosis**[80] are often confused but mean different things:

- **Arteriosclerosis** is the general **hardening, stiffening and loss of flexibility of the arteries** with age. The elastic layer frays and fragments[122]. The connective tissue[81] that surrounds our cells, thickens and calcium gets deposited in this layer, and the muscle in the walls of our arteries gets bigger (hypertrophies), resulting in the hardening of our arteries.
- **Atherosclerosis** is where cholesterol, calcium, and dead cells build up in the artery walls, forming **plaques** that narrow and sometimes block the arteries.

Arteriosclerosis can occur without atherosclerosis, but atherosclerosis only occurs once arteriosclerosis is present.[123]

A Brief History

- In **1833**, Jean Lobstein, a professor working in France[82] who is regarded as the "father of arteriosclerosis"[124], introduced the term **arteriosclerosis** to describe the hardening of the artery walls.
- In **1904**, Felix Marchand, a German scientist[83], first used the word **atherosclerosis** to describe the buildup of fatty plaques inside arteries.[125]

How Atherosclerosis Develops

The process happens slowly over **decades** (the various stages are shown in Figure 12.1):

- **B:** Fatty streaks form on artery walls.
- **C:** These streaks grow into **plaques** (atheroma).
- **D&E:** The plaques get bigger, narrowing the artery.
- **F:** If a plaque **ruptures**, a **blood clot** forms.
- **G:** This clot can completely **block** the artery or **break off**, travelling to another part of the body[84].

---

79 From the Greek word "arteria", meaning artery, and sclerosis, meaning hardening. "Osis" is a Greek suffix that means a diseased condition.
80 From the Greek "athero", meaning gruel, and "sclerosis", meaning hardening, to describe the fatty substance inside a hardened artery. The cholesterol in the walls of arteries literally looks like porridge or gruel.
81 Connective tissue that supports, protects, and gives structure to other tissues and organs in the body. Connective tissue also stores fat, helps move nutrients and other substances between tissues and organs, and helps repair damaged tissue.
82 Professor of Anatomy at Ecole d'obstétrique du Rhin Inférieur (School of Obstetrics of the Lower Rhine).
83 University of Leipzig, Saxony.
84 The medical term for this is embolisation, from the Greek word "embolismos", which means "intercalary" or "interpressure". It also comes from the Greek word "embolus", which means "peg" or "stopper".

Why Is Atherosclerosis so Dangerous?

- In **early stages (A–D)** there are usually **no symptoms**.
- In **later stages (E–G)** symptoms of **heart attacks** and **strokes** occur.

Sometimes, strokes and heart attacks can occur when the atheroma is mild and hard to detect, even with modern tests. This is the likely explanation for **"cryptogenic stroke"** (strokes with no known cause). This process will be explored in more detail in later chapters.

SECTION 5:
13. It is not a Disease of Modern Society

The rise in heart disease in the 20th and 21st centuries has led many to believe that atherosclerosis is a modern condition caused by our lifestyle. However, studies of ancient civilisations prove that this disease has existed for thousands of years.

Ötzi "the Iceman"

Ötzi the Iceman[85], a naturally mummified body from the Copper Age, was discovered in 1991 in the Italian Alps. He lived over 5,300 years ago and was killed by an arrow that ruptured a blood vessel near his shoulder. Despite his physically active lifestyle and a diet considered well-balanced, with low protein and saturated fat[126], Ötzi had severe hardening of the arteries. X-rays of his body showed calcium deposits in his aorta, brain arteries, and leg arteries. He was only around 45 years old and weighed just 38 kg when he died. Modern genetic testing revealed that he had an abnormal chromosome 9, which made him more likely to develop atherosclerosis. Interestingly, DNA studies have found that 19 men currently living in the Alps share his genetic traits.[127]

Ancient Mummies

Evidence of atherosclerosis is not limited to Ötzi. Studies of ancient Egyptian and Chinese mummies, as well as research on the early populations of Peru, Native America, and the Aleutian Islands[86], show that artery hardening was common across different cultures.[128–131] One notable case is Lady Dai, the wife of a high-ranking official in ancient China. She lived around 200 BC and led a wealthy, comfortable life. When her body was discovered, it was found she had been borderline obese, weighing 70 kg at a height of just 1.54 metres (BMI 29.5 kg/m^2). She suffered from high blood pressure, diabetes, and liver disease. An autopsy in 1972 showed that one of her coronary arteries was completely blocked – likely leading to a fatal heart attack at around age 50.[132,133]

Further studies of Egyptian mummies confirm that atherosclerosis was widespread in the past. A 1973 autopsy[87] of an ancient Egyptian mummy, known as PUM II, revealed large plaques in his arteries, with thickening of both large and small blood vessels.[128] In 2009, CT scans of 16 Egyptian mummies found that

---

85 The copper age was from the 5th to 3rd millennium BC. Ötzi was discovered in the Schnalstal/Val Senales Valley, South Tyrol.

86 The Horus Study, Thompson, R.C. et al Lancet 2013: 381(9873)1211–1222.

87 At the Wayne State University School of Medicine in Detroit Michigan.

31% of mummies had clear signs of hardened arteries, while another 25% showed probable signs of the disease.[134] The scans also showed that the condition was more common in those who had lived past 45 years of age, with 87% of older mummies having artery calcification – compared to just 25% of those who died younger.

The Horus study,[130] which examined 137 mummies from four different regions and over 4,000 years of history, found that about 34% showed signs of atherosclerosis.

These studies show that hardening of the arteries is not purely caused by modern lifestyles. While obesity, smoking, and processed foods may have worsened the problem in recent times, atherosclerosis has existed for centuries, even in cultures with mainly vegetarian diets and no tobacco use.

14. Not Just a Disease of Old Age

Many people think hardening of the arteries is a disease that only affects older people because symptoms like heart attacks and strokes usually appear later in life. However, research shows that this condition actually begins much earlier, even in infancy.

A 1953 study,[135] described as a landmark study, examined the arteries of young US soldiers who died in the Korean War. Autopsies found that over 77% of them had signs of coronary artery disease, with some arteries completely blocked. These soldiers were, on average, only 22 years old. This discovery was shocking, but it should not have been had they read previous studies.

Autopsy Studies in the Young

In 1925,[136] a study found fatty deposits in the arteries of babies as young as six months. Fatty streaks, the earliest signs of atherosclerosis, have been detected in infants as young as six months of age.[136–138] By the age of three, nearly every person has the first signs of artery hardening.[139–144] Further studies in Japan and the US[141,145–148] examined young people who had died from accidents or other causes unrelated to heart disease. A Japanese study recorded autopsy results from over 443,000 cases and found that most teenagers already had early signs of hardened arteries.[149] A US study found that 78% of young people, with an average age of just 25, had atherosclerosis. Some even had more than 50% narrowing of their arteries, and in nearly 10% of them, the narrowing was more than 75%. The findings were more severe in Americans than Japanese people of a similar age.[148]

Stillborn Babies

The earliest signs of this disease have even been **found in stillborn babies**, especially if their mothers smoked[150,151] or had high cholesterol.[152]

Progeria

A rare genetic disorder called progeria[88] provides further evidence that atherosclerosis is not just a lifestyle-related disease. The first case of progeria was described in 1886 by Jonathan Hutchinson, a surgeon at the London Hospital.[153] The patient died at 17 years of age.[154] Progeria was then called Hutchinson-Gilford Progeria Syndrome.

---

88 From Greek progeros «prematurely old;» from pro «before, sooner» and geras «old man» The son of Rabbi Harold Kushner suffered from progeria. It prompted Kushner to author a marvellous book called "When Bad Things Happen to Good People" (publisher Schocken Books).

Progeria causes extremely fast ageing. By the age of three years, children with this condition develop severe hardening of the arteries, except the pulmonary artery that takes blood from the heart to the lungs.[155,156] Most die from heart attacks in their teenage years, looking like elderly adults. These children are not overweight, do not smoke, and do not have diabetes, yet their arteries are severely damaged.[157] High blood pressure commences at the age of six years, **well after** they develop severe atherosclerosis of their arteries![158]

Scientists have found that a mutation in these children's DNA creates a mutant protein called progerin that weakens the cells in their artery walls, making them more vulnerable to damage.[159,160] There is hope for these children: the drug Zokinvy (lonafarnib)[89] that suppresses progerin has normalised the life span in mice[161] and has shown promise in patient studies.[162]

The autopsy evidence is irrefutable and the conclusion is inescapable. The risk factors, including high cholesterol, **cannot** be the cause of atherosclerosis.

Contrarian Thought
Medicine considers the start of symptoms, like heart attacks and strokes caused by blocked arteries, as the beginning of the disease.[90] However, these are – like the tip of an iceberg – just the visible effects of the disease atherosclerosis. The truth is that **every person has atherosclerosis from a young age**, without it causing any symptoms.
Atherosclerosis develops long before risk factors currently thought to be the cause, such as obesity, high blood pressure, diabetes, a high cholesterol, and smoking, come into play. While these factors can make the disease worse and increase the chances of strokes and heart attacks after they develop, they cannot, as discussed in Chapter 11, be the cause of atherosclerosis.

Contrarian Thought
The term cryptogenic stroke is used when the cause of a stroke cannot be found. Knowing that there is atherosclerosis from an incredibly early age, one suspects that atherosclerosis is the most likely cause of cryptogenic stroke. The atherosclerosis is severe enough to cause symptoms but not severe enough to be detected by current tests doctors use to look at our arteries. i.e., ultrasound, computerised tomography angiography[91] and magnetic resonance angiography.

89 A specific inhibitor of farnesyltransferase (FTI) was approved for use by the European Medicines Agency in 2022.
90 There are many causes of stroke with blocked blood vessels; atherosclerosis is one of the most common.
91 From Latinized form of Greek angeion – vessel, and graphy from Greek graphia – description of.

15. Elephants and Birds do not Smoke or Eat Meat

Hardening of the arteries happens in all animals to some degree. Unlike humans, animals don't smoke, most don't become obese, and many are herbivores. Interestingly, carnivores, which eat meat and have high-fat diets, are usually lean and show very little hardening of their arteries. This chapter explores the fascinating studies on animal arteries.

In 1939, Herbert Fox[92] from the University of Pennsylvania highlighted the importance of studying animals to understand diseases.[163,164] He noted that hardening of the arteries occurs in most animals, both in the wild and in captivity, and worsens with age, just like in humans. Birds, in particular, develop severe atherosclerosis in the arch of their aorta, an area that experiences strong blood flow due to their powerful hearts – which are 2.5 times heavier than the hearts of mammals with the same body weight. Fox had access to research from the Philadelphia Zoological Society, which had conducted nearly 10,000 animal autopsies over 27 years. His studies revealed that arteriosclerosis is common in animals. He even suggested that because humans suffer from it the most, we might be the least healthy species.

Sylvia Sikes from the University of London studied cardiovascular disease in 201 animals, covering 43 species of mammals and 25 species of birds in Africa.[165] She found early signs of artery hardening in 37 species, mostly in areas of strong blood flow, like the arch of the aorta. She also noticed that in parts of arteries where blood flows smoothly, hardening was minimal.

Dogs and cats, both carnivores, eat high-fat diets rich in cholesterol, yet they don't usually develop atherosclerosis unless their cholesterol reaches extreme levels – far higher than what is seen in humans.[166,167]

For years, scientists believed that strokes did not occur in domestic animals. However, MRI scans have since shown that strokes do happen in animals, but they present differently than in humans. In dogs, for example, a stroke causes them to walk in circles rather than experience paralysis, as seen in people.[168–170]

---

92 Fox wrote Chapter 6 "Arteriosclerosis in lower mammals and birds; its relation to the disease in man" in the same 1933 monograph on atherosclerosis where Anitschow revealed the truth about his rabbit experiments.

16. Physical Damage to the Walls of our Arteries

The idea that atherosclerosis is caused by physical damage to arteries is not new. According to influential German pathologist Karl Albert Ludwig Aschoff,[137] it was Rudolf Virchow (1821–1902) who first examined the histology (microscopic features) of atherosclerosis at the University of Berlin in the 19th century. The first change he observed was loosening of the connective tissue in the inner lining of arteries, the intima. Virchow suggested that this loosening occurred due to increased pressure, causing the plasma (liquid part of blood) to be absorbed into the arterial wall. The connective tissue cells in the wall then enlarged, divided, and formed localised thickenings. Virchow believed inflammation in the blood vessel walls was a secondary response to this process.

As early as 1872, Professor Eduard von Rindfleisch[93] suggested that atherosclerosis develops where arteries experience the most force from blood flow.[171] In a previous chapter, I compared the heart and blood vessels to an irrigation system. Our arteries must handle blood being pumped under high-pressure 60–100 times per minute throughout our lives. This constant force causes wear and tear, leading to the early signs of atherosclerosis long before factors like smoking, obesity, diabetes, or high cholesterol come into play. However, these factors can make the damage worse and cause symptoms to appear earlier.

Two hundred years later, this book makes a very good case for **physical damage to the arteries being the primary cause of atherosclerosis**. Time will tell whether we have managed to convince the scientific community of the validity of this concept.

This chapter explores natural and human experiments that provide strong evidence that physical damage is the main cause of artery hardening.

The Impact of Increased Pressure

With each heartbeat, blood moves through the arteries, pulling on their inner layer (the intima) and straining the elastic and muscular middle layers (media).[121,172-174] Unlike rigid pipes in an irrigation system, arteries can stretch to hold more blood. If someone develops obesity, their body can add up to 3.6 extra litres of blood.[175] Although arteries can expand to handle this at first, they aren't designed for such a high volume. Over time, the increased strain from this extra blood in the circulation damages their walls, making them stiffer. This, together with the increased amount of blood in the circulation, leads to high blood pressure (hypertension).

---

93 Professor of Pathology at Würzburg University.

> **Contrarian Thought**
>
> In appendix B, I have reproduced my hypothesis that atherosclerosis is the cause – not the consequence – of essential hypertension (high blood pressure).

Arteries That Rarely Develop Atherosclerosis

Three arteries in the body generally do not develop atherosclerosis unless they are exposed to higher-than-normal pressure.

1. **Pulmonary Artery:** This artery carries blood from the heart to the lungs. It is exposed to the same cholesterol-rich blood as other arteries but the pressure is much lower[94]. However, in conditions like pulmonary hypertension, where the pressure increases, atherosclerosis can develop.[176]
2. **Internal Mammary Artery**[95] **(IMA):** Located inside the chest wall, this artery is often used in heart bypass surgery because it is resistant to atherosclerosis.[177,178] However, in people with a rare condition called coarctation of the aorta (a severe narrowing or stricture of the body's main artery), the IMA can develop severe atherosclerosis.
3. **The Radial Artery:** Found in the forearm, this artery is also used in bypass surgery because it rarely develops atherosclerosis. One reason may be that it is very straight with few branches, just like the IMA, so it experiences less turbulence.

The Effect of High Pressure on Arteries

In coarctation of the aorta[96], the upper body experiences extremely high blood pressure while the lower body has low pressure. This condition causes severe atherosclerosis in the internal mammary artery but not in other arteries below the narrowing, where blood pressure is lower.[179–182] Not surprisingly, the pulses in the feet of these patients are difficult to locate because of this low pressure.[183]

Animal Studies

Animal studies have shown that when arteries are exposed to higher pressure, they develop atherosclerosis, even in animals on a low-cholesterol diet. Experiments using knockout mice[97] who had a surgically-induced coarctation showed they developed similar changes to those seen in humans with coarctation. The size of the atheromatous plaques above the narrowing increased by a staggering

---

94 12–16mmHg, as opposed to the high pressure of ≥120mmHg in the aorta.

95 Also called the internal thoracic artery.

96 A congenital disorder (condition you are born with) where BP can be as high as 260/120 above and only 100/90 below.

97 A knockout mouse is not a mouse that is KO'd! It's a genetically engineered mouse that has had one or more of its genes turned off. In this study, elimination of the apolipoprotein E (Apo E) gene predisposed these mice to atheroma (plaques).

245% and 145% in male and female mice respectively! There was no increased atherosclerosis below the constriction.[184]

A study was conducted on cingulate monkeys to examine the effects of a narrowed aorta (coarctation). Some monkeys had this condition surgically created, while others did not. They were then fed either a low-cholesterol or high-cholesterol diet. Monkeys with coarctation who ate a low-cholesterol diet developed arteriosclerosis, which is a thickening and stiffening of the artery walls, but they did not develop atherosclerosis. However, monkeys with coarctation who were fed a high-cholesterol diet developed severe atherosclerosis. Interestingly, monkeys without coarctation who ate the same high-cholesterol diet did not develop atherosclerosis.[185]

The Role of Turbulence

Not all arteries under high pressure develop atherosclerosis affecting their walls evenly. It tends to occur more often at branch points where blood flow becomes turbulent. Turbulence adds to the physical stress on artery walls, making them more likely to develop damage and cholesterol buildup. When the inner lining is damaged, gaps open up between the cells, allowing LDL cholesterol to seep into the artery walls.[186] In 1858, Rudolph Virchow from Berlin first discussed shear force, a force that acts parallel to a surface, causing one part of a material to slide past another – essentially attempting to "shear" or cut the material apart.[98][187]

How Veins Respond to High Pressure

Unlike arteries, veins usually have very low pressure. They do not develop atherosclerosis, even though the walls are exposed to the same cholesterol-laden blood as arteries.[188] However, when veins are exposed to high pressure – such as when they are used for heart bypass surgery[99][189] – they begin to develop thickened walls like those seen in early atherosclerosis.[190,191] This suggests that high pressure plays a crucial role in artery disease. The pulmonary veins carry oxygen-enriched blood from the lungs back to the left side of the heart. When the mitral valve on the left side of the heart (see Figure 5.1) is constricted, a condition known as mitral stenosis, it causes high pressure in our pulmonary veins and they develop mild atherosclerosis.[188]

When an artery is surgically connected to a vein, it is called an arterio-venous (A-V) fistula. These fistulas are used when a person's veins are not suitable

---

98 Turbulence and shear stress (the flow of viscous blood over the inner lining of arteries) are discussed in more detail in appendix G.

99 In 1968, René Favaloro from the Cleveland Clinic in Ohio introduced a technique for heart bypass surgery that was widely used for many years. He took a vein from the leg, called the saphenous vein, and connected it to bypass a blocked coronary artery. Initially, these veins were free of atherosclerosis, but once exposed to the higher pressure in the arteries, they began to show early signs of atherosclerosis within three months after surgery. More severe changes developed by the end of the first year. Because of this, surgeons now prefer to use the radial and the internal mammary artery for bypass surgery, as they are more resistant to atherosclerosis.

for inserting a needle and for haemodialysis, a treatment for kidney failure. Because it is connected to an artery, the pressure inside the vein becomes much higher than normal, causing the vein's walls to thicken in a way that resembles arteriosclerosis.[188,192]

When the wall of a vein that is next to and in contact with an artery is subjected to the pulsing of that artery, the wall of that vein develops localised thickening – but the opposite wall where the vein is NOT in contact with the artery is unaffected.[193]

There is one exception: Where the two veins in the legs join together inside the pelvis to form the inferior vena cava (Chapter 5) there is significant turbulence and atheroma develops in 50% of us.[194,195]

Experimental Evidence of Physical Damage

Studies on animals[196–197] have shown that when arteries experience direct trauma, they develop lipid (fat) deposits in the walls, similar to atherosclerosis. In humans, artery damage begins in childhood, long before cholesterol buildup starts. Over time, repeated injury leads to inflammation and scarring, creating the plaques seen in atherosclerosis.

Contrarian Thought – The Main Cause of Atherosclerosis

While factors like obesity, diabetes, high cholesterol, and smoking make the condition worse, the root cause appears to be the relentless force of blood against artery walls. The two most important things to prevent atherosclerosis are avoiding weight gain and not smoking. Obesity is particularly harmful as it increases pressure inside arteries. Smoking is even worse because it damages the artery lining, making it easier for cholesterol to build up.

---

17. Eliminating Atherosclerosis and Insights from World War II

When doctors study diseases with unpredictable outcomes, they use a method called a randomised trial. This means only half the participants receive the treatment being tested, allowing researchers to compare results.

In an unexpected way, a real-life randomised study on nutrition took place during World War II. In the later years of the war, severe food shortages affected countries like West Germany,[199,200] Finland,[201] Sweden,[202] and Norway,[203] while southern Germany and Switzerland had plenty of food.[199–201,203] In areas with shortages, people were eating as little as 1,000 to 1,200 calories a day, similar to some modern extreme diets.

In Switzerland and southern Germany where food was still available, obesity, heart attacks, and strokes continued during and after the war. The average cholesterol level in southern Germany was about 230 mg/dL (5.95 mmol/L). However, in countries with food shortages, people lost a lot of weight. Young adults weighed around 58 kg for women and 62 kg for men. Their cholesterol levels dropped from 230 to 140 mg/dL (5.95 to 3.62 mmol/L), and there were no recorded deaths from heart attacks or strokes.

Autopsies in West Germany at the time found little to no advanced atherosclerosis. Between 1945 and 1948, there were no recorded cases of death from heart attacks or severe artery blockages, compared to both pre-war (1939) and post-war (1955) records. Similar findings were observed in Rotterdam, Netherlands.[200] A similar pattern had also been seen after World War I.[204]

Starving prisoners of war had mostly smooth, healthy arteries with little atherosclerosis.[199] However, after the war, when people started eating normally again, obesity returned, cholesterol levels increased, and smoking became more common. As a result, deaths from coronary artery disease rose dramatically – from 2,600 in 1948 to 24,000 just four years later, and 38,000 fifteen years after the war ended.[200]

Shortly after the war, a 1947 autopsy study in New York examined over a thousand individuals and found that atherosclerosis was twice as common in people with obesity compared to those who were undernourished. Those with average nutrition had more atherosclerosis than the undernourished but less than the obese.[205] Other studies found that people who lost a lot of weight before death had less fat buildup in their arteries[205], and poorly nourished people with an addiction to alcohol also had less atherosclerosis.[205] Additionally, patients with cancer who experience weight loss often had fewer signs of atherosclerosis compared to patients without cancer.[206]

These remarkable findings seem to have been forgotten or overlooked.
Marked weight loss resulted in the normalisation of cholesterol
and the disappearance of atherosclerosis,
the major cause of heart attacks and strokes.

Although living on just 1,200 calories a day would be difficult, the only sure way to eliminate atherosclerosis completely would be to become extremely thin. The question remains as to whether moderate weight loss can also reverse atherosclerosis. Studies have shown that lifestyle changes[207] and weight loss surgery[208] can partially reduce it, but no study has shown complete reversal.

In Summary
While extreme weight loss may eliminate atherosclerosis, even moderate weight loss can help reduce obesity-related risks such as diabetes, high blood pressure, and high cholesterol. Ideally, we should aim for a BMI of 25 kg/m² or lower to improve our overall health.

18. Cholesterol and Hardening of our Arteries

> **This chapter will, but should not be, controversial.**

Because cholesterol builds up in artery walls, many assume it must be the main cause of atherosclerosis. This idea is known as the "cholesterol hypothesis." The European Atherosclerosis Society strongly supports this view, stating that many clinical and genetic studies clearly show LDL cholesterol causes atherosclerotic cardiovascular disease (ASCVD).[209]

However, their official statement is more cautious, saying that cholesterol-rich LDL and other similar lipoproteins *are involved* in the development of ASCVD – but they do not say LDL is the *main* cause.

Saying that LDL cholesterol is *not* the primary cause of atherosclerosis might seem radical, but I am not alone in questioning this idea (see Appendix G). This does not mean high LDL cholesterol *doesn't* worsen atherosclerosis – it does. However, it does so by passively collecting in artery walls that are already damaged, rather than starting the process itself. Similarly, lowering cholesterol can reduce the risk of heart attacks and strokes, at an individual level, only slightly, but at a community level, the benefit is enormous. This is discussed further in Chapter 20, *Understanding Benefit*.

Similar, severe atherosclerosis is found at autopsy in patients aged 16–65 with and without elevated cholesterol.[210]

> **Contrarian (But Not Original) Thought**
>
> The main cause of atherosclerosis is physical damage to artery walls, not cholesterol. When arteries are damaged, cholesterol builds up inside them through various mechanisms.

There are other theories about what causes atherosclerosis, but none fully explain why it mostly affects only parts of arteries – blood vessels exposed to high pressure. It is a complex topic, and for those interested, Appendix G provides a more detailed discussion.

SECTION 6:
Understanding Benefit and Causation vs Association

"There are three types of lies: lies, damn lies, and statistics."
– Benjamin Disraeli (1804–1881), British Prime Minister

"If your experiment needs a statistician, you need a better experiment."
– Ernest Rutherford (1871–1937), British physicist

"Most people use statistics like a drunk man uses a lamppost: more for support than illumination."
– Andrew Lang (1844–1912), Scottish author

"Statistics are never a substitute for common sense."
– Amit Kalantri (1988–), Indian author

"Statistics cannot be any smarter than the people who use them. And in some cases, they can make smart people do dumb things."
– Charles Wheelan (1966–), American author, professor, speaker, and political reformer

"To call in the statistician after the experiment is done may be no more than asking him to perform a post-mortem examination: he may be able to say what the experiment died of."
– Sir Ronald Fisher (1890–1962), "The father of statistics"

"I can prove anything by statistics except the truth."
– George Canning (1770–1827), English statesman

As you can see, there has always been a great deal of scepticism about statistics. However, when used correctly – which is unfortunately not always the case – statistics are a vital part of all research.

This section will explain the difference between relative and absolute risk and the distinction between association and causation. These are two crucial concepts that help to clarify why so much confusion exists, particularly in the popular press.

I hope medical reporters will read this chapter and use it to ask researchers the right questions, ultimately providing better information for their readers.

19. Association versus Causation

Studies known as 'observational studies' are widely used in medical research. There are two main types of observational study. One is called a *case-control study*, where researchers compare people who have a disease to people who do not have it to find possible causes for that disease. The other type, a *cohort study,* follows a group of healthy people over time to see who develops the disease and what lifestyle factors might be linked to it.

However, just because two things are associated does not mean one causes the other. A great example of this is peptic ulcer disease (ulcers in the stomach or small intestine). Observational studies once suggested that stress, personality type, smoking, alcohol, aspirin, and spicy foods caused peptic ulcers. However, Australian doctor Barry Marshall and his pathology colleague Dr Robin Warren discovered that a bacterium called Helicobacter pylori was the real cause. It took years to convince the medical community of this. To prove his point, Dr Marshall even gave himself an ulcer by swallowing the bacteria! They were awarded the 2005 Nobel Prize for Medicine for their discovery.

Observational studies have also led to some strange claims, like:
- eating more nuts makes you live longer.[211]
- eating eggs prevents diabetes.[212]
- eating just one egg a week could be enough to lower your risk of dying from heart disease.[213]
- eating chilli peppers more than four times per week decreases the risk of death.[214]
- eating avocados[215] or drinking coffee lowers the risk of heart disease.[216]

There is no way these claims could be true for someone who smokes, is severely overweight, has high blood pressure, diabetes, and high cholesterol.

If the same link is found repeatedly in different studies, and the connection is very strong, it is more likely to be real. This was the case with smoking – studies showed that smokers had much higher death rates than non-smokers, mainly due to heart attacks and lung cancer.[217]

Meta-Analysis

A common research method is *meta-analysis*, where results from multiple studies are combined. This can lead to findings from huge numbers of patients, making them seem more reliable. However, not all studies are high quality, and mixing poor-quality research with good research does not improve it.[218] Just like adding a rotten apple to a barrel of fresh apples doesn't make the rotten one good!

A meta-analysis does not prove cause and effect; it only measures how strong an association is. To be reliable, it must use strict rules to make sure all studies included are of similar quality. However, many meta-analyses have later been proven wrong by large, well-run studies.[219]

If you see words like *associated with*, *linked to*, or *tied to*
in a scientific paper or news article,
remember that these words only describe a connection.
They do *not* prove one thing causes another.

20. Understanding Benefit – A Chocolate Bar vs a Motor Car

A 50% discount might sound like a huge benefit, but it makes a big difference whether that discount is on a $2 chocolate bar or a $100,000 car. A 50% discount on the chocolate bar saves just $1. But if everyone in a town of 200,000 people bought a half-price chocolate bar, the total savings in that town would be $200,000. The relative reduction benefits the community as a whole (how much is saved in total).

A 50% discount on the car saves $50,000. But if only one person bought a half-price car, the savings would still be just $50,000. The absolute reduction benefits the individual (how much you save personally).

Understanding Risk Reduction in Medicine

In medicine, the effectiveness of treatments is measured in three ways:

- **Relative Risk Reduction (RRR):** This is the percentage difference in risk between people who receive treatment and those who don't. It tells us how much a treatment reduces risk compared to doing nothing. This shows us how much a treatment will benefit society overall – just like the discount on a chocolate bar can benefit a lot of people.
- **Absolute Risk Reduction (ARR):** This measures the actual difference in how many people experience an adverse outcome, comparing those who take the treatment and those who don't. Like the actual dollar amount you save on a purchase, ARR tells us how much a treatment benefits an individual.
- **Numbers Needed to Treat (NNT):** This tells us how many people need to be treated for just one person to benefit from that treatment.[220,221] If fewer people need to be treated for one person to benefit (i.e. the NNT is lower), it means the treatment is more effective. A high NNT means the treatment isn't very effective for individuals.

These terms are important when looking at cholesterol-lowering drugs, discussed in Appendix E, and high blood pressure, discussed in Chapter 31.

When Risk is High, Fewer Patients Are Needed

If a disease is deadly, we need to study fewer patients to see whether a treatment works. For example, before antibiotics, tuberculosis (also known as the "white plague") caused 120 deaths per 100,000 people. When the first antibiotic, streptomycin, was introduced, deaths dropped to just 14 per 100,000 – a huge reduction![222]

Similarly, when British sailors suffered from scurvy on long voyages due to a lack of vitamin C, it only took a study of 12 sailors to prove that eating limes prevented scurvy. Interestingly, the sailors who ate rats did not suffer from scurvy because rats naturally produce their own vitamin C![223]

Comparing Two Studies on Blood Pressure Treatment

Let's look at two different studies on high blood pressure treatment:

- The **Veterans Administration (VA) Study**[224] in 1967 looked at 143 men with very high blood pressure, diastolic blood pressures averaging 115 through 129 mm Hg. These patients were at serious risk, so it didn't take many people to show a clear benefit. This study found a **71.5% relative risk reduction (RRR)**, and a **27.5% absolute risk reduction (ARR)**. Only **2.29 patients** needed to be treated for one person to benefit.
- The **Medical Research Council (MRC) Study**[225] looked at 17,354 people with mild high blood pressure. Since their risk of ASCVD was lower, the study needed more patients to show a smaller benefit. The **RRR was 2.55%**, and the **ARR was just 0.14%**. In this case, **143 people** had to be treated for one person to benefit.

Even though the benefit to individuals in the MRC study was small, the impact on society could still be massive. In the US, **116 million people** have high blood pressure. If they all took medication and the annual ARR was only 0.14%, it would still prevent **over 2 million strokes and heart attacks**. This shows that even a small benefit to individuals can lead to big benefits for society because the RRR, the benefit to society is 2.5% – just like the chocolate bar vs motor car example.

Confidence Intervals: How Certain Are the Results?

Scientists use statistics to determine whether a treatment actually works. A study's results include a statistic called a **confidence interval (CI)**, which shows that there is a range of possible outcomes. For example, if a treatment has a **relative risk of 0.70**, this means the treatment reduces risk by about **30%**. If you see the confidence interval written as **95% CI: 0.65–0.96**, it means the researchers are **95% sure** the real benefit is somewhere between **4%** (1.0 minus 0.96) and **35%** (1.0 minus 0.65). The closer the two numbers are, the more reliable the result. If the confidence interval is **more than 1.0**, it means the study **failed** to prove the treatment works.

Key Takeaway

When looking at medical studies, it's important to understand the difference between relative and absolute risk reduction. A treatment might have a small benefit for individuals but still have a huge impact on public health. And while statistics help prove whether treatments work, it's always important to check how reliable the results really are.

STRUCK DOWN BY THE GODS

SECTION 7:
Types of Strokes

Strokes can occur when a blood vessel in or on the surface of the brain either bursts or becomes blocked.

The symptoms we experience largely depend on which part of the brain is affected.

Strokes caused by ruptured blood vessels are more likely to cause a severe headache and, if they are large enough, can rapidly lead to reduced consciousness.

This section describes the different types of strokes that can occur due to either a burst or blocked blood vessel.

21. Strokes Due to Blocked Blood Vessels

A stroke caused by a blocked blood vessel happens when a blood clot prevents blood from reaching the brain. This type of stroke is called an ischaemic stroke. Blood clots can form from problems with blood clotting in different areas, including:

- the heart
- the large arteries in the neck (carotid and vertebral arteries)
- the arteries on the surface of the brain
- tiny blood vessels deep inside the brain (lacunar strokes)
- veins that drain blood from the brain.

When a blood clot forms in one part of the body and travels through the bloodstream to block an artery elsewhere, this is called an embolism. The concept of embolism was first described by French physician Jean-Baptiste de Senac in 1749,[226] but it wasn't widely accepted until German physician Rudolf Virchow's research in 1860.[227]

Sometimes, strokes can happen in areas of the brain that don't cause noticeable symptoms.[228] These "silent strokes" can only be detected using brain scans like CT (computed tomography) or MRI (magnetic resonance imaging).[229] The three main causes of ischaemic strokes are:

1. blood clots from the heart due to an irregular heartbeat called atrial fibrillation
2. atherosclerosis (narrowing of the large arteries to the brain due to fatty deposits), and
3. blockages in tiny blood vessels deep in the brain, known as lacunar strokes.

However, in 20–30% of cases, doctors cannot find a clear cause for a stroke.[230,231] This is called a cryptogenic stroke.

Figure 21.1. A drawing of the heart showing diseases that can cause a blood clot to form, travel to our brain and cause a stroke. The term 'left atrial myxoma' refers to a tumour that can grow inside the chamber of the heart[7] Reproduced with Permission Elsevier.^

^ From: Rights and Permissions (ELS) <Permissions@elsevier. com> Date: Sat, 28 June 2025, 12:41 am Subject: Re: Copy of 250613-006213: Permission to reproduce an illustration Y [250409-004647] [250627-021430]

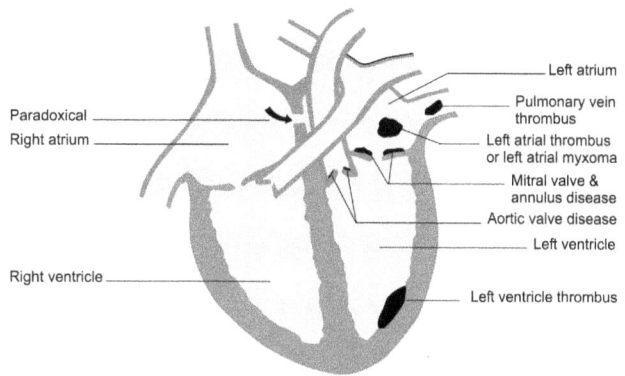

Labels: Paradoxical, Right atrium, Right ventricle, Left atrium, Pulmonary vein thrombus, Left atrial thrombus or left atrial myxoma, Mitral valve & annulus disease, Aortic valve disease, Left ventricle, Left ventricle thrombus

Heart Conditions and Stroke

Certain heart conditions (Figure 21.1) increase the risk of stroke by causing blood clots to form in the heart and travel to the brain. The most common is atrial fibrillation (AF), where the heart's small chambers beat irregularly, allowing blood to pool and form clots.

Other conditions, including heart valve disease, tumours in the heart (such as atrial myxoma), and structural abnormalities like a patent foramen ovale (a small hole between the heart's chambers that should close after birth but remains open in some people), can also lead to strokes. Atrial fibrillation is discussed in more detail in Chapter 35. The other conditions shown in Figure 21.1 are covered in Appendix C.

Doctors use sound wave tests called echocardiograms to check for heart problems. A transthoracic echocardiogram (TTE) involves placing a probe on the chest to take images of the heart. A more detailed test, the transoesophageal echocardiogram (TOE/TEE in the US), involves inserting a probe down the throat to the food pipe (oesophagus) to capture clearer images of the heart. TOE is more effective at picking up abnormalities such as heart valve infections (endocarditis), atrial myxoma, and a patent foramen ovale.[233]

Atherosclerosis and Stroke

In the early 20th century, doctors believed strokes were caused by spasm of the brain's blood vessels. However, in 1905, pathologist Hans Chiari from Prague observed blood clots on atherosclerotic plaques (fatty deposits) in the carotid arteries of stroke patients. This finding suggested these clots could travel to the brain and cause a stroke.[234] This idea was not widely accepted until 1951 when Canadian-born neurologist C. Miller Fisher provided strong evidence linking strokes to atherosclerosis of the carotid artery[100].[235,236]

Atherosclerosis can cause severe narrowing and even total blockage of the carotid arteries, increasing the risk of stroke. Strokes from disease of the carotid arteries and its branches are usually large (Figure 21.2) and result in significant disability. Stroke can be prevented by surgery called carotid endarterectomy that removes fatty plaques from the carotid artery. While carotid artery disease is more common in Caucasians, narrowing of the arteries inside the brain (intracranial stenosis) is more common in people of Asian descent.[237–239] Sometimes, instead of a blood clot forming, pieces of the fatty plaques (cholesterol) can break off and travel to the brain, blocking blood flow and causing a stroke. These cholesterol emboli can block the blood vessel in the eye, causing temporary or permanent

---

100 It was not easy to change doctors' minds. It took the journal two years to accept and finally publish his paper! Miller Fisher listened very carefully to his patients and was seen doing autopsies at all hours of the day and night. He saw a patient who told him he went blind in the right eye and yet weak down the left side of his body. Miller Fisher knew that the internal carotid artery supplied blood to the eye and brain on the same side. You may recall that one side of our brain controls the opposite side of our body. Miller Fisher was the first to describe temporary blindness in one eye as a warning symptom of stroke.

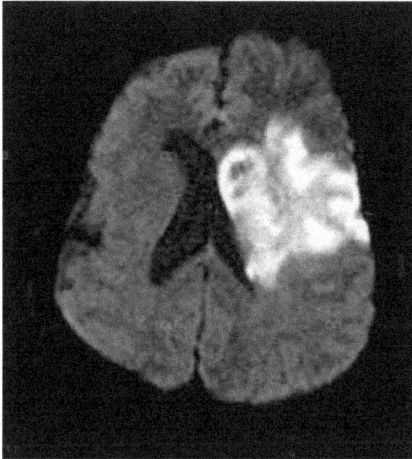

vision loss in that eye. Doctors can see these when they use a special instrument called an ophthalmoscope to look in the eye.

Figure 21.2. An MRI scan showing a large stroke (the white area) in the part of our brain supplied by the middle cerebral artery, a branch of the internal carotid.

Blockage of Small Blood vessels

Lacunar strokes occur when tiny blood vessels deep inside the brain become blocked (Figure 21.3). These strokes are usually caused by long-term high blood pressure or diabetes, which lead to scarring and thickening of the blood vessel walls.[101][240] Lacunar strokes are small (less than 15 mm in diameter), but if they affect a critical part of the brain, they can still cause serious disability.

The term "lacune" was first used in 1838 by Amedée Dechambre, an intern at the Salpêtrière Hospital in Paris.[241] In the 20th century, Miller Fisher helped to establish the link between these tiny blockages and strokes.[242,243] In Western countries, lacunar strokes account for 15–25% of all ischaemic strokes.[244–246] Most people recover well from a lacunar stroke, but in some cases, the damage can be significant.

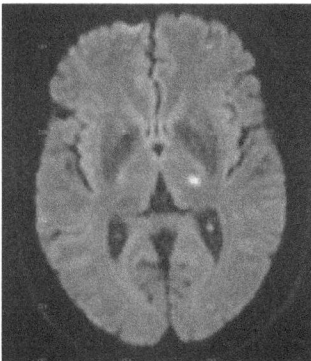

Figure 21.3. An MRI scan showing a lacunar stroke.

---

101 Lipohyalinosis is the term used to describe what happens when blood vessel walls in the brain are replaced by scar (fibrin) tissue. Scavenger white blood cells are filled with the breakdown of blood (cholesterol and protein).

22. Strokes Due to Ruptured Blood Vessels

Strokes caused by burst blood vessels are called haemorrhagic strokes[102]. This chapter explains the types of strokes that happen when a blood vessel bursts. Intracerebral haemorrhage is bleeding **inside** our brains. Bleeding can also occur **outside** our brains in the layers or spaces between the brain and the skull (Figure 22.1).

The number of strokes from bleeding blood vessels has dropped a lot thanks to better treatment for high blood pressure. Back in 1977, when I was training as a neurologist, we would see two or three cases of large brain haemorrhages each week in the autopsy room.

However, in the future, strokes from burst blood vessels may increase. As we age, our blood vessels weaken because a protein called amyloid builds up in their walls. This condition, called cerebral amyloid angiopathy (CAA), makes bleeding more likely. With people living longer, more of us may develop CAA-related bleeding.

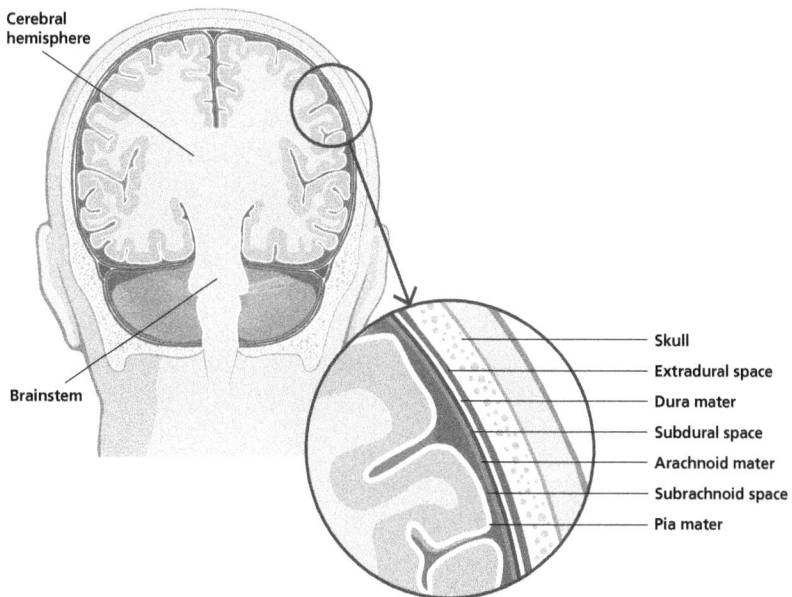

Figure 22.1 The layers or spaces between the skull and the brain.
Illustration Sandra Coventry.

---

102 From Latin haemorrhagia, "bleeding violently," from haima "blood" (see -emia) + rhage "a breaking," from rhegnynai "to break, burst."

The hard bone of our skulls encloses and protects our brains. Inside the skull, our brain is surrounded by three layers of tissue called the meninges.[103]

1. A thick, leathery outermost layer called the dura mater.[104]
2. A delicate middle layer called the arachnoid mater.[105]
3. A thin, innermost layer called the pia mater[106] that covers the surface of our brains.

Bleeding can occur between:

- the pia mater and arachnoid mater – called a subarachnoid haemorrhage.
- the arachnoid mater and dura mater – called a subdural haemorrhage.
- the dura mater and the skull – called an extradural haemorrhage.

The subarachnoid space contains the cerebrospinal fluid (CSF), which can be removed for testing with a lumbar puncture. Strictly speaking, subdural and extradural haemorrhages are not classified as strokes, but they can cause paralysis mimicking a stroke.

Blood Clots Outside the Brain

Although extradural and subdural haemorrhages are not regarded as strokes, they are included in this chapter for completeness.

Extradural Haemorrhage

An extradural haemorrhage[107] happens between the skull and the dura mater. It can occur after a severe head injury and skull fracture that causes an artery to burst. Because arteries carry blood under high pressure, a large blood clot can form quickly. If not treated with emergency surgery, this condition is usually fatal.

A famous case is Natasha Richardson, daughter of actress Vanessa Redgrave, who died from an extradural haemorrhage hours after a skiing accident in Quebec.

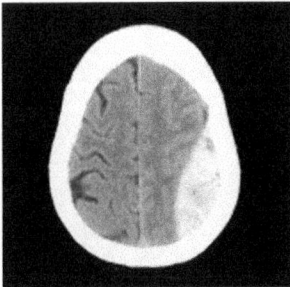

Ancient humans in France,[247] Greece,[248] and Peru[249] performed a type of skull surgery known as trepanation[108] to remove such blood clots. Some of these procedures were done for medical reasons, while others had spiritual or ritual significance[109].

Figure 22.2. A large extradural haemorrhage. The haemorrhage is typically convex towards the brain.

---

103 Greek: membrane.
104 Latin: tough mother .
105 As it resembles a spider's web.
106 Latin: tender mother.
107 Called epidural in the United States.
108 From the Greek word trypanon, meaning augur or borer.
109 The history of trepanation can be found at https://thereader.mitpress.mit.edu/hole-in-the-head-trepanation/.

Subdural Haemorrhage

A subdural haemorrhage (Figure 22.3) occurs beneath the dura mater and outside the arachnoid membrane. It results from a burst vein, so bleeding happens slowly under low pressure. Older people may not notice symptoms because their brains shrink with age. This creates more space for a blood clot to form without causing immediate pressure. A subdural haemorrhage can be triggered by even a minor head injury, and sometimes it happens without any known injury.

Blood thinners like Coumadin (warfarin) and the newer anticoagulants[110] can increase the risk of subdural haematomas. Other risk factors include conditions that affect blood clotting, like leukaemia, liver disease, or a low platelet count. Repeated small bleeds over weeks or months can lead to a chronic subdural haematoma.

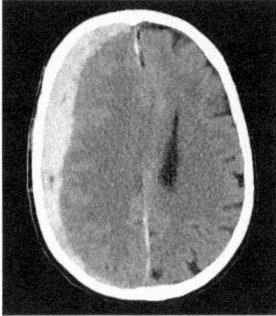

Figure 22.3. Subdural haemorrhage or haematoma. The haemorrhage is concave towards the brain, the classical feature of a subdural haematoma.

Subarachnoid Haemorrhage

A subarachnoid haemorrhage (SAH) happens when an artery bursts, causing high-pressure blood to rush into the space beneath the arachnoid layer (Figure 22.4). This bleeding can be deadly in about one-third of cases.[250] Another third of patients who survive the initial bleeding may die within hours or days if the bleeding happens again or complications arise.

The most common cause of SAH is a ruptured aneurysm, which is a weak, balloon-like bulge in an artery. These aneurysms are often called "berry aneurysms" because they look like small berries. The aneurysm shown in Figure 22.5 results from a congenital problem[111]. They tend to form in areas where arteries branch.

The first operation to treat a brain aneurysm was performed in 1885 by British physiologist and neurosurgeon Sir Victor Horsley.[251] He tied off the internal carotid artery in the neck, taking advantage of the circle of Willis – a network of arteries that helps supply blood to the brain even if one artery is blocked.

---

110 Known as novel oral anticoagulants (NOACs), these drugs inhibit the mechanism that causes our blood to clot. They include the direct thrombin inhibitors dabigatran and ximelagatran and the factor Xa inhibitors rivaroxaban and apixaban.

111 Congenital refers to a condition that is present at birth. These are different to conditions that are inherited, hereditary or familial, which are passed down through generations. Congenital problems that are not in the family can occur. Not all familial problems are obvious at birth. Relatives can inherit a tendency to develop them many years later, as happens with berry aneurysms.

One major breakthrough in brain medicine was cerebral angiography, invented in 1927 by Portuguese neurologist Antonio Egas Moniz[112]. This technique allows doctors to see blood vessels using a special dye. Today, safer methods like CT angiography (CTA) and magnetic resonance angiography (MRA) have mostly replaced traditional angiography.

Antonio Moniz was a scientist and doctor with many interests. He was the first Portuguese person to win a Nobel Prize. He received this award in 1949 for a controversial procedure called a lobotomy (or leucotomy), which was used to treat severe mental illness. This operation involved cutting the connection between the frontal lobe and the rest of the brain.

The idea for this procedure is believed to have come from the case of Phineas Gage. In 1848, Gage suffered a terrible accident when a steel rod went through his cheek and damaged the front part of his brain, known as the frontal lobe. His doctor, John Martyn Harlow, noticed that Gage's personality changed a lot after the accident. Previously friendly and responsible, Gage became impulsive, bad-tempered, and had poor judgment. Today, Harvard University displays the steel rod that injured him and a cast of his skull.

Another famous case involving a lobotomy was that of Rosemary Kennedy, the sister of Robert, Edward, and John F. Kennedy. She had a mild intellectual disability, and in 1941 her father arranged for her to have the procedure because he was embarrassed by her interest in boys. Sadly, the operation left her with severe mental and physical disabilities[113]. She lived until the age of 86, but her father never told the family what he had done.

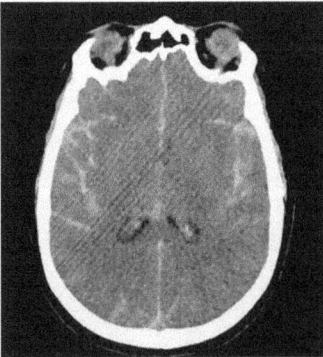

Figure 22.4. Subarachnoid haemorrhage. The blood fills the gyri (valleys) formed by the natural folds of the brain.

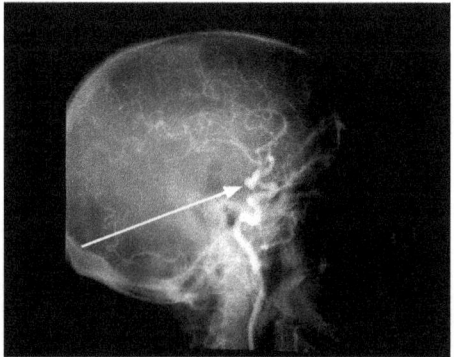

Figure 22.5. An Angiogram with an aneurysm (arrow) on the anterior cerebral artery.

---

112 1874–1955.

113 The operation failed and Rosemary lost most of her ability to walk or talk. Her personality was altered forever. After being released from the hospital, Rosemary was immediately placed in an institution.

Giovanni Battista Morgagni[114] is often credited as the first person to describe a cerebral aneurysm.[252] However, he only suggested that such a condition might exist. The first actual description of an unruptured aneurysm came from Francesco Biumi.[115] In 1765, he discovered it during an autopsy on a 52-year-old woman.[253]

In 1780 Sir Gilbert Blane[254] reported the first clinical description of a ruptured aneurysm. Sir Gilbert is better known for his reforms in naval hygiene. He was a physician at St. Thomas' Hospital and physician-in-ordinary to King George IV and King William IV. In 1779 he accompanied Admiral

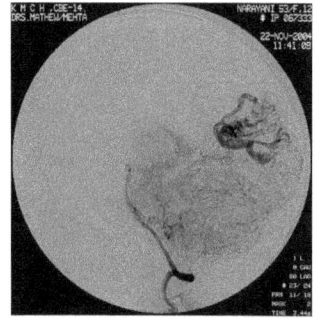

Figure 22.6. An angiogram (x-ray of Blood vessels) showing a large arteriovenous malformation (AVM).

(later Lord) Rodney to the West Indies as his private physician. On the expedition, Blane enforced the use of lemon juice and other fresh foods in the diet. In doing so he prevented scurvy.

The principal treatment of SAH is to prevent recurrent bleeding. This is achieved by finding the cause and doing something about it as early as possible.

Berry aneurysms are the main cause of a SAH, but they can also be caused by arteriovenous malformations (AVMs) – which are bundles of malformed blood vessels. AVMs are extremely rare, affecting one in every 100,000 people.[116] They resemble a clump of pulsating worms. Large arteries and veins are directly connected without any of the smaller blood vessels in between. This means the blood enters veins under a higher pressure making them vulnerable to rupture. Despite this increased pressure, bleeding from an AVM is rare. AVMs were recognised in ancient Egypt as early as 1500 BC.[255]

Blood-thinning drugs such as warfarin can lead to a SAH,[256] but the risk is less with the novel oral anticoagulants (NOACs).[257] Subarachnoid haemorrhage can occur with a low platelet count (thrombocytopaenia) – remember the platelets are the tiny cells that stick together to start blood clot formation to prevent bleeding.[258] Drugs that prevent platelets from sticking together are called antiplatelet agents. These include aspirin, clopidogrel (Plavix), ticagrelor (Brilinta), and dipyridamole (Persantin). There is a very small increased risk of intracerebral, subarachnoid[259,260] and subdural haemorrhage[261] when these drugs are used in isolation. The risk increases (as does the benefit) when they are used in combination[262], and especially when they are used with blood thinners such as warfarin and the NOACs.

---

114   Professor of Anatomy at Padua.
115   Professor of Anatomy in Milan.
116   A statistic for expressing incidence rates, which are the number of new cases of a condition during a certain time period.

Tiny haemorrhages called cerebral microbleeds are sometimes seen on MRI scans. They do not cause symptoms, so patients do not know they have them. However, these microbleeds do increase the risk of bleeding into the brain, so people who have them cannot take blood thinners.

A 1983 review of the literature undertaken by this author found 123 different proven causes of SAH. There were 18 different brain tumours; 31 abnormalities of blood vessels; eight infections and nine abnormalities of the clotting mechanism.[263] The American musician, actor, director, screenwriter, and producer Bret Michaels suffered a SAH, and Kamimura Ukyou (Kami), the drummer from visual kei band Malice Mizer, died from a SAH.

Blood Clots Inside the Brain

Bleeding with High Blood Pressure

A blood clot inside the brain is called an intracerebral haemorrhage (or ICH; noting the cerebrum is the brain). This is what most people would recognise as a stroke. ICH can occur anywhere in the brain and accounts for approximately 15% of all strokes.[264] In patients with high blood pressure, ICH can occur deep inside certain parts of the brain (Figures 22.7 & 22.8). Many Famous people have died of an intracerebral haemorrhage, including actor Cary Grant, and the American-born Afro-French dancer, singer, and actress Josephine Baker, who was variously nicknamed the "Bronze Venus," the "Black Pearl," and the "Créole Goddess".

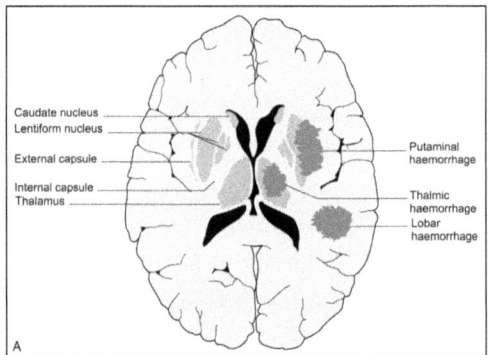

Figure 22.7. Sites of bleeding into the cerebral hemispheres (the large part of the brain). Image gifted to the author by H.J.M.Barnett.

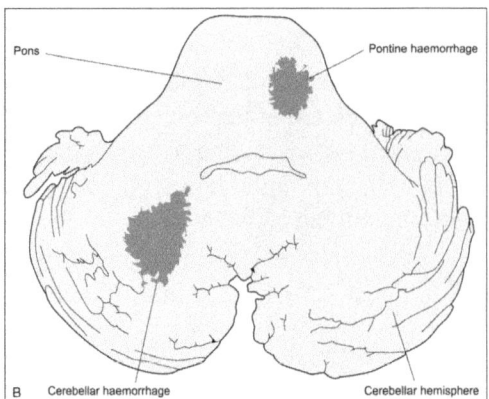

Figure 22.8. Sites of bleeding into the brainstem (the stalk of the cauliflower described in the chapter on the brain), the cerebellum and the small parts at the back of the brainstem). Image gifted to the author by H.J.M.Barnett.

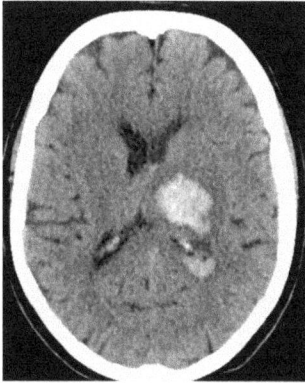

Figure 22.9. Hypertensive intracerebral haemorrhage in the basal ganglia deep inside the brain.

Traditional teaching is that ICH related to high blood pressure is caused by rupture of a tiny bubble on a very small blood vessel deep inside our brain. These bubbles are called Charcot-Bouchard aneurysms, named after two French doctors who described them: Professor Jean-Martin Charcôt and his colleague Charles-Joseph Bouchard from the Saltpêtrière Hospital in Paris Later in their professional lives these men fell out. They had a dispute about nominating Dr Joseph Babinski for a professorship.[265] Babinski was Charcot's preference, but Bouchard won and Babinski was not appointed. Babinski is remembered to this day for the reflex that bears his name. The Babinski reflex is tested by scratching the sole of the foot. If the big toe points down, this is a normal reflex; if it moves up it is abnormal, indicating a problem in the brain or spinal cord.

Whether Charcot-Bouchard aneurysms actually exist has been challenged, with some suggesting that the coils and twists in tiny blood vessels were misinterpreted as aneurysms. Either way, rupture of these very tiny blood vessels can cause an ICH.

Bleeding with Cerebral Amyloid Angiopathy

The second most common cause of ICH is a condition called cerebral amyloid angiopathy (CAA). This causes bleeding just beneath the surface of the brain. These haemorrhages are referred to as "lobar haemorrhages" (Figure 22.10). The blood vessels in our brains become more fragile with advancing age

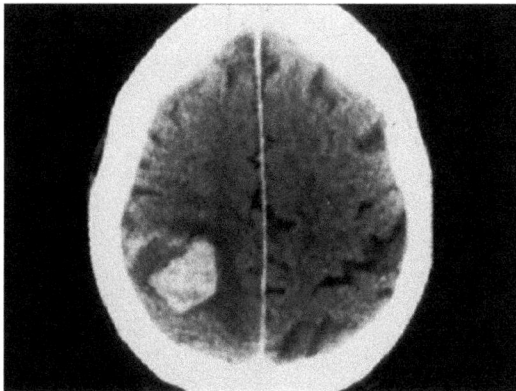

as a protein called amyloid (different to the amyloid plaques seen with Alzheimer's) builds up in their walls. The vessel wall is weakened and becomes prone to rupture.[266] At this stage it is not clear why amyloid occurs more frequently in the later years of life. Haemorrhage due to hypertension and CAA accounts for nearly 90% of all cases of ICH.[264]

Figure 22.10. Intracerebral haemorrhage due to cerebral amyloid angiopathy (CAA). The amyloid seen in the brain with Alzheimer's disease is different to that in CAA.

Blood-Thinning Drugs

The third leading cause of ICH is blood-thinning medication. These drugs, such as warfarin, help prevent blood clots in the heart and blood vessels. The discovery of warfarin is an interesting story. During the Great Depression, farmers in North America noticed their cattle were dying from internal bleeding after eating mouldy hay.[267] This condition was called "sweet clover disease." About ten years later, a Wisconsin farmer named Ed Colson took a dead cow and a bucket of blood that wouldn't clot to an agricultural research station. After six years of study, scientist Karl Link and his team discovered that a natural blood thinner called coumarin was in the hay. When coumarin was exposed to mould, it turned into dicoumarol, which stopped blood from clotting.

The **W**isconsin **A**lumni **R**esearch **F**oundation funded Link's work and patented the drug, naming it 'warfarin' after their foundation. Later, Link also developed a rat poison using warfarin. Despite its reputation as "rat poison," doctors started using warfarin as a medication. In 1955, US President Dwight Eisenhower was given warfarin after a heart attack!

Warfarin became widely used in the 1960s and was very effective at preventing blood clots in the lungs (pulmonary embolism); far fewer people died.[268]

However, early on, doctors had trouble measuring how thin a patient's blood was, which sometimes led to excessive bleeding. In the 1980s, the World Health Organization introduced the prothrombin time international normalisation ratio (PT INR) test, which made warfarin safer by standardising the dosage.[269]

Rarer Causes of Bleeding into Our Brains

Other rare causes of ICH include drug use, particularly use of amphetamines, cocaine, and ecstasy. Brain tumours can also cause bleeding, especially aggressive cancers like glioblastoma multiforme (a very aggressive brain tumour) and melanomas that go to the brain. The most common cancers that spread to the brain and cause bleeding come from the lungs, skin, placenta, and kidneys.

Intraventricular Haemorrhage

The brain has four fluid-filled spaces called ventricles. Sometimes, bleeding can happen inside these spaces. This is called an intraventricular haemorrhage (IVH) (Figure 22.11). IVH is very rare and usually caused by high blood pressure, aneurysms, malformed blood vessels[117] (AVMs), or premature birth.

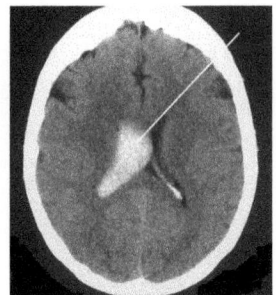

Figure 22.11. Intraventricular haemorrhage. The blood is filling and hiding the right ventricle. By convention, the left side of a CT scan is actually the right side of the image.

---

117 AVM: arteriovenous malformation.

SECTION 8:
Symptoms and Warning Signs of Stroke

This section discusses the warning symptoms a small number of people may experience, indicating the possibility – but not the certainty – of a stroke.

For most of us, the only warning signs are ageing and the development of obesity, often complicated by high blood pressure (hypertension), diabetes, and elevated cholesterol.

It also explores the symptoms that may occur if a stroke happens, and describes medical conditions that can cause similar symptoms to those of a stroke.

The warning signs of a stroke caused by a blocked blood vessel are the same as those of an actual stroke, except that they go away by themselves (see **FAST** below).

23. Warning Symptoms of Stroke

Most people who have a stroke don't get a clear warning. The only signs might be health problems that increase the risk, like obesity, high blood pressure, smoking, diabetes, and high cholesterol. However, there are some mild symptoms that can be early warnings of a serious stroke.

Stroke Caused by a Ruptured Blood Vessel

Bleeding in the Brain

If a blood vessel bursts and causes bleeding in the brain (called an intracerebral haemorrhage), there is usually no warning. The main risk factor is having high blood pressure (BP) that hasn't been properly managed. Current World Health Organization recommendations and European guidelines are to aim for a BP of 140/90 or lower,[270,271] whilst in the US it is 130/80 or lower.[272]

Subarachnoid Haemorrhage (SAH)

SAH is bleeding outside the brain, in the fluid that surrounds it. About 30–40% of people with SAH may have a sudden, severe headache days, weeks, or even months before the main bleed happens. This is caused by a small leak in a weak spot of a blood vessel (an aneurysm), known as a sentinel[273] bleed.

A sentinel bleed headache is extremely painful, reaching its worst point within five minutes. This is called a thunderclap headache. It might affect just one part of the head or spread all over. Other symptoms include nausea, vomiting, sensitivity to light, and sometimes neck pain or stiffness. Loss of consciousness is rare, but can happen. Unfortunately, some people ignore these warning headaches.

Another possible warning sign occurs when an aneurysm grows larger and presses on a nerve that controls the eyelid and eye movement. This can cause a 3rd nerve palsy resulting in a drooping eyelid, double vision, and a larger pupil.

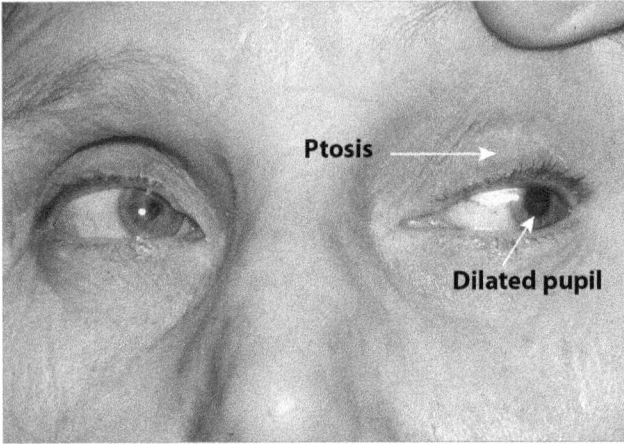

Figure 23.1. A left 3rd nerve palsy (paralysis) with a droopy eyelid (held up to reveal the pupil) and a dilated (enlarged) pupil, with the eye turning outwards. Ptosis is a drooping eyelid.

Stroke Caused by a Blocked Blood Vessel

In about 15% of strokes caused by blocked blood vessels, people experience warning signs called transient ischaemic attacks (TIAs), also known as "mini-strokes." There has been considerable debate about the definition of a TIA. At the 1985 4th Princeton conference, the term TIA was <u>arbitrarily</u> adopted to describe symptoms that went away by themselves within 24 hours.[274] MRI scans can pick up signs of a stroke as early as 30 minutes after symptoms start.[275] Once symptoms have lasted 60 minutes, only a tiny proportion (<2%) will disappear within 24 hours.[276]

If someone has a TIA, their risk of a full stroke within the next 90 days is about 10–20%,[277–279] with most happening within the first two days.[280] However, most people who have a stroke don't have a warning TIA.

A TIA happens when blood flow to part of the brain is temporarily blocked. Symptoms appear suddenly and are at their worst immediately or within minutes. They usually last between 2–15 minutes before going away. However, very rarely symptoms can get worse over time, either by getting more intense or spreading to more parts of the body[118]. This often leads to an incorrect diagnosis of migraine. How to tell the difference between a TIA and a migraine is discussed in Chapter 25.

Recognising and acting on these warning signs can help prevent a more severe, disabling, or even life-threatening stroke.

---

118 These mainly occur when the blockage affects a tiny blood vessel inside the brain.

24. Symptoms of Stroke

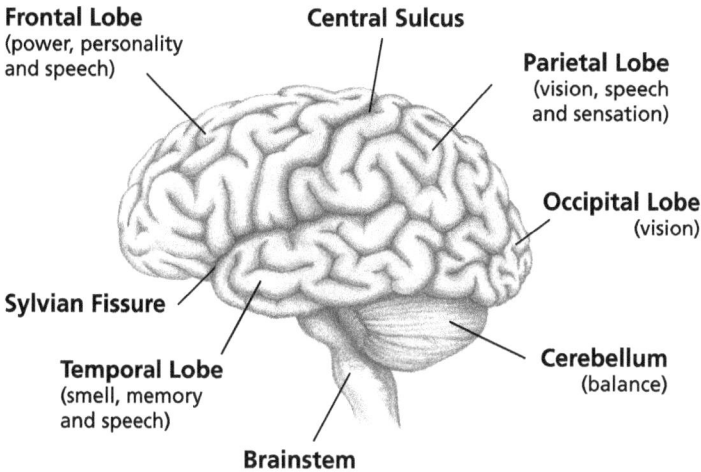

Frontal Lobe
(power, personality
and speech)

Central Sulcus

Parietal Lobe
(vision, speech
and sensation)

Occipital Lobe
(vision)

Sylvian Fissure

Temporal Lobe
(smell, memory
and speech)

Cerebellum
(balance)

Brainstem

Figure 24.1. A view of the left side of the brain showing the frontal, parietal, occipital, and temporal lobes of the cerebral hemispheres, the brainstem and the cerebellum. It shows the various functions controlled by these areas of the brain. The brain looks like a lot of rolling hills with gullies (sulci or fissures) between them. It could also be described as two "bunches of cauliflower" (the hemispheres and cerebellum) attached to a stalk (the brainstem). The brainstem is like a highway for electrical messages, carrying signals between the brain and the rest of the body through the spinal cord. The **central sulcus** separates the frontal lobe from the parietal lobe, while the **Sylvian fissure** separates the frontal and parietal lobes from the temporal lobe. Despite its complex structure, the brain is actually very soft to the touch. Illustration: Sandra Coventry.

This chapter explains the different symptoms of a stroke. Several things influence which symptoms a stroke will cause, including:
- Which part of the brain is affected (Figure 24.1).
- Whether the stroke affects the back of the brain (occipital lobe) or one of the eyes – determines if and how vision is affected.
- Whether we are right or left-handed – which affects how speech is disturbed.
- Whether the stroke happens in part of the brain supplied by a large artery on its surface (Figures 5.2–5.4), a small blood vessel deep inside the brain or, very rarely, a vein that drains blood away from the brain.

A stroke resulting from a burst blood vessel (haemorrhage) or a blocked artery can cause the same symptoms if the same brain area is affected. However, haemorrhagic strokes also cause a rapid increase in pressure inside the skull, which can lead to vomiting, drowsiness, or even a coma. Headaches are more common with a haemorrhagic stroke than with a stroke caused by a blocked artery.

Stroke Symptoms Based on Brain Area

The most common type of stroke happens in the arteries that supply the hemispheres of the brain, as they carry 90% of the blood to the brain[119].

- **Frontal lobe:** Causes weakness on the opposite side of the body, mostly in the face and arm. If the stroke is on the left side, the ability to speak is often affected (called dysphasia). If it's on the right side, speech may be slurred.
- **Occipital lobe (back of the brain):** Causes vision loss on the opposite side of the body. If the eye itself is affected, there may be partial or total blindness in that eye.
- **Parietal or temporal lobe:** May cause loss of sensation on the opposite side of the body. Depending on which side is affected, it can also lead to speech problems or an unawareness of having had a stroke.
- **Cerebellum:** Causes clumsiness in the arm or leg on the same side of the body.

Right or Left-Handed

Doctors ask if someone is right or left-handed because speech is controlled by the left side of the brain for 90% of right-handed people and about 50% of left-handed people. If a stroke affects speech (beyond slurred speech), it's likely happened on the left side of the brain, which is called the dominant hemisphere. The other side is called the non-dominant hemisphere. In left-handed people the right hemisphere is dominant, the left non-dominant.

Thunderclap Headache

A thunderclap headache is an extremely painful headache that happens immediately or worsens within 5 minutes.[281] It is often a sign of a burst blood vessel in the brain, called a subarachnoid haemorrhage (SAH). Similar headaches can occur during physical exertion or sexual activity, and the key differences between these and a dangerous SAH headache are covered in the next chapter.

Weakness or Paralysis

A stroke often causes weakness or paralysis. When this occurs, it mainly affects the face and arm, sometimes the leg, on the opposite side of the damaged part of the brain. A brain tumour in the same area could cause similar symptoms. However, stroke symptoms happen suddenly, while tumour symptoms develop slowly over months to years. The exception is blockage of tiny blood vessels inside the brain. Stroke symptoms can come on over minutes spreading slowly from one part of the body to other parts of the body.

---

119   Only 10% is carried by the vertebral arteries to the brainstem and cerebellum.

Another way to check for a stroke is the **STR test**:
- **S (Smile):** One side of the face may be drooping.
- **T (Talk):** Speech may be slurred, or the person may struggle to say a simple sentence.
- **R (Raise arms):** One arm may be weak, or the person may not be able to lift it.

A similar method, originally developed in Cincinnati, called the Cincinnati Prehospital Stroke Scale[282], is **FAST**[120].
- **F**ace: Look for weakness of the face
- **A**rm: Look for weakness of the arms
- **S**peech: See if speech is affected, and
- **T**ime: Refers to acting quickly, because more brain cells die as time passes without treatment.

Both these methods, and the many others developed, detect stroke in close to 90% of patients.[283] In this chapter we will discuss the symptoms of strokes that can be detected and those that can be missed.

Speech Problems

A stroke can cause different types of speech issues:
- **Dysarthria:** Slurred speech, similar to being drunk.
- **Dysphasia:** Difficulty forming or understanding words.
- **Aphasia:** Total loss of speech (but still able to make sounds[121]).

Non-fluent (Broca's) dysphasia: The person knows what they want to say but struggles to get the words out, similar to a severe stutter. This happens when the stroke affects the dominant (most often the left) **frontal lobe**. It is usually accompanied by weakness in the face and arm on the opposite side of the body to the side of the brain affected.

Fluent dysphasia: Speech flows easily but with incorrect or mixed-up words.
- Someone may replace letters within words[122] (e.g., saying "hat" instead of "cat").
- Others may replace entire words[123] (e.g., saying "drive" instead of "car").
- If the **parietal lobe** is affected, a person may struggle to name objects despite knowing what they are. This is called nominal dysphasia.
- If the **temporal lobe** is affected, speech may become completely mixed up, e.g., saying "jumped over horse the lazy dog" instead of "the horse jumped over the lazy dog"[124]. They may also invent words[125]. This is called **Wernicke's dysphasia** and can make the person seem confused.

---

120 A modification of FAST is FASTER: Face, Arm, Stability, Talking, Eyes (double vision or loss of vision) and React (call emergency ambulance).
121 Mutism, or the inability to make sounds, is never caused by a stroke.
122 Called literal paraphasic error.
123 Called verbal paraphasic error.
124 Referred to as 'word salad', as if all the words were thrown into a bowl and mixed up.
125 Called a neologism, from ancient Greek neos, meaning "new," and logos, meaning "word".

Vision Problems

A stroke can cause vision loss or double vision.

Vision Loss

- If a blood clot blocks the artery to **one eye**, there may be complete or partial blindness in that eye. Vision loss often starts as a curtain dropping over the eye. A transient ischaemic attack (TIA or "mini-stroke") can cause this type of temporary visual loss for minutes or longer[126].
- If a stroke affects the **occipital lobe**, it causes vision loss to the opposite side of both eyes. The person may only see one half of objects.
- Some people develop **cortical blindness**, where both occipital lobes are damaged, and they don't realise they are blind[127].
- If a stroke affects the right side of the brain, causing vision loss to the left, the person may not notice[128] they can't see to the left. This can lead to confusion, like walking past a door they were looking for because it was on the left.

Double Vision

Double vision alone is rarely, if ever, a sign of stroke. A common cause is a "lazy eye" or squint. However, if a small blood vessel in the **brainstem** is blocked, it can cause double vision only when looking to the side opposite to the damage (Figure 24.2).

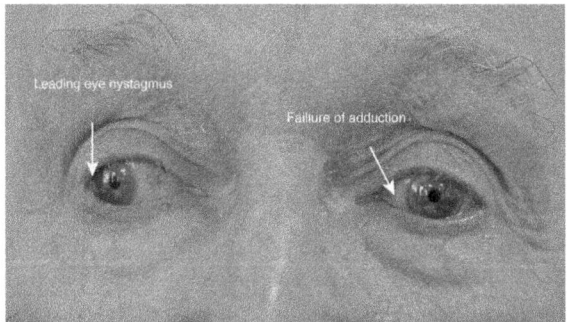

Leading eye nystagmus

Failure of adduction

Figure 24.2. An example of double vision caused by a stroke. The left eye is not able to move past the midline (failure of adduction), while the right eye displays jerky movements called nystagmus.

Dizziness, Vertigo, and Unsteadiness

Dizziness, also called giddiness, is a vague symptom. If dizziness is the only symptom, it is very unlikely to be caused by a stroke. It is usually due to problems with the inner ear's balance system or low blood pressure.

Vertigo, a feeling that the room or head is spinning, can sometimes happen during a stroke, but only if the stroke affects the brainstem or cerebellum (the small part

---

126 Referred to as Amaurosis fugax, from the Greek "amaurosis," meaning dark, and the Latin "fugax," meaning fleeting.
127 Known as Anton syndrome or visual anosognosia.

of the brain behind the brainstem). Feeling light-headed or faint is <u>not</u> a symptom of stroke.

A stroke in the cerebellum can cause vertigo, clumsiness in the arm and leg on the same side, and slurred speech. However, some people with cerebellar strokes do not have vertigo. Instead, they may feel extremely sick, vomit a lot, and struggle to stand up. If you cannot stand while vomiting, this suggests a problem in the cerebellum rather than a stomach issue. In rare cases, vomiting can be so severe that it causes bleeding in the oesophagus (gullet), a condition called haematemesis.

If a stroke affects the brainstem, symptoms may appear on both sides of the body. Slurred speech, difficulty swallowing, double vision[129] (objects appearing side-by-side or on top of each other), and weakness on one or both sides can occur.

Other causes of vertigo, not related to stroke, will be discussed in the next chapter.

Numbness and Pins and Needles

Feeling pins and needles or numbness in one part of the arm or leg is not usually a sign of a stroke. However, a "pure sensory stroke" (a stroke that only causes sensation changes) can happen suddenly, affecting the face, arm, leg, and torso equally.[284]

Some people confuse a stroke with a heart attack because they have heard that heart attacks cause symptoms in the left arm. A heart attack causes pain in the arm, chest, neck, shoulder, or jaw, shortness of breath, and sweating. However, stroke does not cause pain or shortness of breath.

Strokes That Only Others Notice

A stroke in the non-dominant parietal lobe (usually the right side of the brain) can happen without the person realising it. They may not notice vision loss on the left or even be aware of severe weakness in their left arm and leg[130]. In rare cases, they might not recognise their own arm or leg when shown to them[131].

If the stroke is mild and does not affect walking, the person may seem confused or "lost" in their own home. They ignore everything on their left side. A typical example is the person who wants to go to the bathroom, they walk down the hallway and miss the toilet on their left side. They then turn around and see it because it is on their right-hand side. This can be difficult for inexperienced doctors to diagnose.

---

129 Called diplopia, from two Greek words: diplous, meaning double, and ops, meaning eye.
130 Called anosognosia.
131 Called autotopagnosia, from the Greek a and gnosis, meaning "without knowledge", topos meaning "place", and auto meaning "oneself".

Can a Child Have a Stroke?

Most people are shocked to learn that strokes can happen at any age, including in children as young as one year old. Though rare, stroke affects between 1.3 and 13 per 100,000 children per year. In a city of five million people, this means 65 to 650 children may have a stroke each year. The causes of stroke in children are different to those in adults.[285]

Seek Urgent Medical Help

If you or someone you know has any of these symptoms, seek medical care immediately. The best place to go is a major hospital with a dedicated stroke unit and team. In some cities, stroke ambulances are equipped with a CT scanner and can start treatment before arriving at the hospital.

> The faster treatment is commenced, the better the chances of recovery.

25. No, We are Not Having a Stroke

This chapter talks about medical conditions that can seem like a stroke. These are divided into problems affecting the head and neck and those affecting the arms and legs.

Head and Neck Symptoms

Bell's Palsy (Facial Paralysis)

One of the most common conditions mistaken for a stroke is Bell's palsy, which causes paralysis on one side of the face. The exact cause is unknown.

A simple way to tell the difference between a stroke and Bell's palsy is to look in a mirror and try to raise your eyebrows. If you cannot wrinkle your forehead on the affected side, it is Bell's palsy. Other symptoms may include increased hearing in one ear and a change in taste.

There is no specific cure, but steroid tablets (cortisone) can help reduce swelling and speed up recovery.[286] It is also important to protect the eye on the affected side by taping the eyelid shut and using artificial tears to keep it moist.

Vertigo (Spinning Sensation)

Vertigo is the feeling that either one's head or the room is spinning. While it can be a symptom of a stroke in the brainstem or cerebellum, stroke-related vertigo always comes with other symptoms like slurred speech, double vision or weakness of the face or limbs.

If vertigo happens on its own, it is almost never due to a stroke. Instead, it is usually caused by problems in the inner ear or the nerve connecting the ear to the brain.

Labyrinthitis and Vestibular Neuronitis

Labyrinthitis and vestibular neuronitis cause severe vertigo with nausea, and vomiting. People with labyrinthitis may also experience hearing loss, but those with vestibular[132] neuronitis do not. The vertigo is still present when lying perfectly still with the eyes closed, and even the slightest movement of the head makes it much worse. The vertigo lasts days to weeks, gradually subsiding.

Benign Paroxysmal Positional Vertigo (BPPV)

BPPV is type of vertigo that happens only when the head is moved, e.g. looking up, bending over, or moving the head quickly. Episodes last about 20–30 seconds and go away when you stop moving. It is treated with specific head exercises, like the Brandt-Daroff exercises or the particle repositioning manoeuvre.

---

132 The vestibular nerve is the nerve that conveys messages about balance from the ear to the brain. It is one half of the vestibulocochlear nerve; the cochlear half conveys hearing messages.

Ménière's Disease

Ménière's disease causes severe vertigo, nausea and vomiting that lasts for hours. Transient hearing loss may occur during an episode, and if it does this confirms the diagnosis – because this only occurs with Ménière's and nothing else[133]. Over time, repeated attacks can lead to permanent hearing loss. Eating too much salt can trigger episodes, so avoiding salty foods is recommended.

Double Vision

Double vision by itself is virtually never a sign of a stroke. Most cases of isolated double vision especially when tired, are caused by a lazy eye, also called strabismus or squint.

A very rare stroke in the brainstem can cause double vision with one object next to the other but only when looking in one direction, not the other. This is due to blockage of a very tiny blood vessel affecting the pathway[134] that connects the muscles of the eyes to each other and to the balance mechanism in the ear (the labyrinth). This is a type of lacunar stroke that was described in the previous chapter.

Blackouts (Loss of Consciousness)

Blackouts do not happen with strokes. They are usually caused by either epilepsy or an irregular heartbeat.

Epileptic Seizures

Minor seizures: There are two types of minor seizures that can cause "blackouts", the first is called an absence seizure[135]. A person suddenly stops responding, stares into space for 15–30 seconds, and then continues as if nothing happened. They are not aware that they are having a seizure. Young children having this type of seizure are often thought to be daydreaming, and often the diagnosis is not made for several years. The second type of minor seizure is called a complex-partial seizure[136]. Here the patient stares into space and is unresponsive. There may be warning symptoms[137] such as déjà vu, a strange smell or taste (usually unpleasant), or a rising sensation in the stomach. Some people may fidget or lick their lips during this type of seizure. The person is confused for a few minutes afterwards.

Major seizures: The person falls to the ground, loses consciousness, their limbs stiffen and then they convulse. They may bite their lip or tongue and lose control of their bladder and/or bowel. This is the tonic-clonic seizure[138].

---

133 The medical term for this phenomena is pathognomonic, from Greek pathognōmonikos 'skilled in diagnosis', from pathos 'suffering' + gnōmōn 'judge'.
134 The median longitudinal fasciculus.
135 Previously called petit mal.
136 Previously called temporal lobe epilepsy, but we now know that they do not all arise in the temporal lobe.
137 Called auras.
138 Previously called grand-mal.

Stokes-Adams Attacks

A Stokes-Adams attack is when the heart briefly stops[139] beating, causing a sudden blackout. The episode is short and there are no abnormal movements. This is treated by inserting a pacemaker.

Migraine Aura Without Headache

Migraine aura without headache is where people experience migraine symptoms without the headache.

Symptoms can include tingling in the face, arm, or leg, speech problems, and even temporary paralysis or unconsciousness. Many people only have the typical vision disturbances that happen with migraine, including flashing lights, zig-zag lines[140] or even patches of missing vision[141]. The clue is that in migraine these move across or enlarge to affect more of the vision.

These symptoms can seem like a stroke, but they usually start gradually and move from one part of the body to another. For example, tingling may start in the hand, then spread up the arm, and finally affect the face and leg. By the time it reaches the foot, the tingling in the hand has disappeared. Early symptoms improve before the next symptom occurs or reach peak severity, which never happens in a stroke – making it a clear way to tell the difference.

Arm and Leg Symptoms

Saturday Night Palsy

Saturday night palsy happens when a person falls asleep with their arm hanging over the armrest of a chair, putting pressure on a nerve in the upper arm. When they wake up, they have a droopy wrist and cannot lift their wrist or fingers backwards.

It is called Saturday night palsy because it often happens after drinking too much and falling asleep in a chair. Although a stroke can cause arm weakness, it never causes a wrist drop.

Carpal Tunnel Syndrome

Carpal tunnel syndrome is a common nerve problem that causes numbness and tingling in the thumb, index, middle, and part of the ring finger. It often wakes people up at night, and symptoms improve if they shake their hands or lift them above their head.

Unlike a stroke, carpal tunnel symptoms go away with movement. They can also happen during activities like driving, typing, cycling or using tools.

---

139 Called complete heart block.
140 Called photopsia, from the Greek words phos (φως) meaning "light" and opsis (όψις) meaning «sight». It literally means «seeing light».
141 Called scotomata, from Late Latin scotoma, from Latinized form of Greek skotōma "dizziness," from skotoun "to darken," from skotos "darkness" (from PIE root *skoto- "dark, shade.").

Foot Drop

Foot drop occurs when the nerve just below the knee[142] is squashed, coming on during sleep. It causes an inability to lift the foot and often, but not always, numbness between the first and second toes. The foot drop can last hours to weeks and goes away on its own but the person may need to wear a splint to prevent tripping while walking.

Key Takeaways
Bell's palsy affects the face and can be distinguished from a stroke by checking if you can wrinkle your forehead.
Vertigo alone is not a stroke, and it is usually caused by problems in the inner ear.
Double vision alone is never due to stroke.
Blackouts do not happen in strokes – they are usually caused by seizures or heart problems.
Migraines without headaches can mimic strokes, but the symptoms move gradually from one part of the body to another, with the initial symptoms have lessened or gone before the later symptoms appear or worsen.
Saturday night palsy and carpal tunnel syndrome cause arm problems but are not related to stroke.
Foot drop can happen from sleeping in a bad position but never with a stroke.

These conditions can seem like a stroke, but they have clear differences. If in doubt, seek medical help.

---

142 The common peroneal or common fibular nerve.

SECTION 9:
Risk Factors

Stating the Obvious Is Not a Contrarian Thought
The autopsy evidence is irrefutable, the logic is valid, and the conclusion is inescapable.
Autopsies show that atherosclerosis begins decades before the onset of risk factors and is present in 100% of people by the age of three. Therefore, these risk factors cannot be the primary cause of atherosclerosis.
Twenty-seven per cent of patients with ST-elevation myocardial infarction (or STEMI, a type of heart attack) have none of the well-known risk factors.[113]
Between seven and twenty per cent of stroke patients do not have any of the so-called risk factors.[287–290]
These risk factors help identify which people are at risk of developing symptoms related to atherosclerosis, not of strokes caused by other things (such as heart or blood conditions). In general (but not always), these symptoms occur in people with more severe atherosclerosis. Once risk factors develop – particularly smoking and obesity, with its complications of high blood pressure, elevated cholesterol, and diabetes – they make the condition worse. Risk factors are discussed in this section.

Risk Factors

Risk factors are medical conditions we develop and lifestyle choices we make that indicate that we are at increase our risk of stroke and heart attack. Some risk factors – such as increasing age, gender, ethnicity, and, in a small number of cases, inherited genetic factors – are beyond our control. These are referred to as **non-remediable (or non-modifiable) risk factors**.

Remediable or Modifiable Risk Factors

These are risk factors we can do something about. They include:
- Obesity
- Hypertension (high blood pressure)
- Diabetes
- Cigarette smoking
- Physical inactivity
- Alcohol misuse
- Hyperlipidaemia (elevated cholesterol)

- Asymptomatic carotid stenosis (narrowing of the main artery in the neck)
- Atrial fibrillation (irregular heartbeat)

The **major risk factors** are increasing age, smoking, and obesity.

Despite decades of awareness, a 2023 study of 20 to 44-year-olds in the US found that an increasing number of people are developing obesity-induced hypertension, diabetes, and elevated cholesterol.[291]

This section discusses how we can estimate our risk of stroke using the **Atherosclerosis Cardiovascular Disease (ASCVD) Risk Estimator**. Other risk assessment methods are outlined in *Appendix D*.

Modifying Our Lifestyle and Risk Factors

Current Recommendations:

- Lose weight and aim for a **body mass index(BMI) of 20–25 kg/m²** or a waist circumference of (measured 1 cm above the belly button) of < 50% of our height.
- **Quit smoking.**
- Aim for a **blood pressure of <140/90 mmHg** (US: <130/80 mmHg).
- Follow a diet **low in saturated fat, high in fibre, and containing fish**.[143] US guidelines recommend a **plant-based or Mediterranean-style diet**, rich in vegetables, fruits, nuts, whole grains, lean vegetable or animal protein (preferably fish), and vegetable fibre.
- Engage in **3.5–7 hours of moderate physical activity per week** or **30–60 minutes most days**.
- If diabetic, aim for an **HbA1c of <7%** (US: <6.5%).[292]
- Lower LDL cholesterol with **a high-intensity statin** (a dose expected to reduce LDL by ≥50%), targeting **serum LDL <70 mg/dL (3.89 mmol/L)**. If LDL remains high despite statin use, consider adding **ezetimibe** or using it as an alternative if statins are not tolerated.

The **first two recommendations – losing weight and quitting smoking – provide the greatest benefits**.

Significant weight loss can lower blood pressure, reduce cholesterol, and potentially eliminate diabetes. The effects of smoking on stroke risk are discussed in a later chapter. Extreme weight loss, as observed during World War II, has been shown to completely eliminate the atherosclerosis that causes strokes and heart attacks.

These recommendations are aimed at reducing the risk of stroke and heart attack caused by atherosclerosis – the leading cause of heart attacks and some strokes.

However, some stroke causes, including **atrial fibrillation (an irregular heartbeat), a heart defect (e.g., a hole in the heart), rarer stroke causes (outlined in Chapter 23), and strokes due to ruptured blood vessels**, are only minimally influenced by modifying these risk factors, aside from controlling blood pressure.

---

143 In this book, I argue that this might be a contentious recommendation.

26. Estimating our Risk

The American College of Cardiology and the American Heart Association (ACC/AHA) used to have a tool to estimate the 10-year risk of developing heart disease, stroke, or poor circulation in the legs (atherosclerotic cardiovascular disease or ASCVD)[144]. However, this tool was found to overestimate risk and has now been replaced by the PREVENT risk estimator[145], which uses different factors to assess risk. This is shown in Table 26.1.

	10-Year-Risk of ASCVD Symptoms					
Risk Factor	50		60		70	
	Male	Female	Male	Female	Male	Female
Age	1.5%	1.1%	2.8%	2.1%	5.9%	4.7%
High Blood Pressure*	2.6%	2.0%	4.7%	3.7%	8.3%	6.8%
Diabetes*	2.8%	2.3%	5.0%	4.1%	8.7%	7.3%
High Cholesterol*	2.4%	1.6%	4.7%	3.0%	8.9%	5.6%
The Full Monty**	19.3%	17.1%	22.6%	18.9%	26.4%	20.8%

Table 26.1. The ACA/AHA PREVENT Risk Estimator Plus4. BMI set at 25 for calculations. *These figures represent the risk when this is the only risk factor. The numbers used in these calculations are: Isolated systolic high blood pressure 160. Isolated high cholesterol, total 240(6.21mmol/L), HDL 40(1.03mmol/L). The Full Monty refers to high systolic BP of 160 on treatment, total cholesterol 240mg/dL(6.21mmol/L), HDL 40mg/dL(1.03mmol/L), on a statin, diabetes, and current smoker.

Increasing age has the greatest impact on the risk of stroke and heart disease, as damage to blood vessels increases over time. By age 70, the risk is about four times higher than at age 50. Other factors like high blood pressure, high cholesterol, and diabetes each increase the risk by about 1.5% each.

At age 50, having all four major risk factors, i.e. high blood pressure, diabetes, high cholesterol, and smoking – can increase the risk by 14 to 16 times.

The PREVENT risk estimator allows people to calculate their personal risk. Other methods for assessing cardiovascular risk are discussed in Appendix D[146].

---

144 The risk estimator is not suitable once we have already had symptoms of ASCVD.
145 https://professional.heart.org/en/guidelines-and-statements/prevent-calculator.
146 The appendices and references are located at: https://www.understandingneurology.com.au/books/struck-down-by-the-gods.

If we suffer a TIA or minor stroke, within 5 and 10 years the cumulative incidence (the overall chance of getting a disease or condition over a period of time) of stroke is 12.5%[147] and 19.8%[148] respectively.[293] The risk is highest in the first year after the TIA or minor stroke; 5.94%[149] in the first year, 1.8%[150] per year in the second through fifth years, and 1.72%[151] per year in the sixth through tenth years.

The increased risk of cardiovascular disease (in asymptomatic individuals) with increasing levels of total cholesterol using the American Heart Association PREVENT™ Online Calculator is shown in Table 26.2. As you can see the difference between the lowest level of total cholesterol and the maximum level is 0.08% per year over 10 years and 0.15% per year over 30 years.

Total Cholesterol mg/dL (mmol/L)	% 10-year-risk	% Annual risk	% 30-year-risk	% Annual risk
130 (3.4)*	1.2	0.12	7.2	0.24
150 (3.9)	1.3	0.13	7.6	0.25
200 (5.2)	1.5	0.15	8.7	0.29
250 (6.5)	1.7	0.17	9.9	0.33
300 (7.6)	1.9	0.19	11.2	0.37
320 (8.3)**	2.0	0.20	11.8	0.39

Table 26.2 The 10-year, 30-year-risks and annual % risks with increasing levels of total cholesterol. *minimum amount permitted, **maximum amount permitted. Calculations are for a 50-year-old man, systolic blood pressure 120, BMI 25, eGFR 140, HDL 100 without diabetes, smoking, or on lipid lowering agents (the UACR, HBA1c and zipcode not incorporated into the calculations).

---

147 95%CI, 11.0%–14.1%.
148 95%CI, 16.7%–23.1%.
149 95%CI, 5.18–6.76; 38 studies; I2 = 97%.
150 95%CI, 1.58–2.04; 25 studies; I2 = 90%.
151 95%CI, 1.31–2.18; 12 studies; I2 = 84%.

27. Choosing our Parents

The title of this chapter might seem strange since we can't choose our parents. Doctors often ask if there is a family history of stroke or heart attack, assuming that if a close relative has had one, we might have inherited "bad genes." However, lifestyle plays a huge role. For example, my mother died of a stroke in her 50s, suggesting a possible abnormal gene may have caused the stroke. In reality, she had the "full monty" of risk factors: she was severely overweight, with diabetes, high blood pressure, and she smoked. Her health issues were likely more due to lifestyle choices than genetics.

Atherosclerosis, the stiffening and cholesterol buildup in the walls of the arteries, affects everyone to some degree, from a very young age and worsening with age. Some people develop symptoms while others don't, which explains why some have a "positive" family history of stroke or heart attack while others don't.

Only a few genes are linked to a higher risk of stroke. Genes are stored in our 46 chromosomes, which are made of DNA$_{152}$. Each of us inherits half our DNA from each parent. In 1953, scientists James Watson and Francis Crick described the double-helix structure of DNA,[294] earning them the 1962 Nobel Prize$_{153}$. They questioned the current beliefs at that time$_{154}$ and saw what others had missed, including Rosalind Franklin, whose research was crucial to this discovery. Sadly, she passed away in 1958 and did not receive the Nobel Prize.

Some genetic factors do increase stroke risk. The Ötzi iceman, for example, had a chromosome 9 abnormality that led to severe early atherosclerosis.[295] About 20–30% of people inherit a tendency for atrial fibrillation, a major cause of stroke.[296] Others inherit a condition called familial hypercholesterolemia (FH), which leads to high cholesterol and a greater risk of heart attack or stroke. Many different gene variants have been associated with FH.[297] However, these genetic conditions account for only a small percentage of cases.

Stroke is more common in identical$_{155}$ compared to non-identical$_{156}$ twins, suggesting a possible genetic link.[298–300] Studies of identical twins show that many have similar patterns of artery disease affecting the arteries to their hearts, suggesting a genetic influence.[301] There is a single case report of similar findings in non-identical twins.[302]

---

152 DNA deoxyribonucleic acid.
153 On 27 November 1895, Alfred Nobel finalised his will and testament, leaving most of his wealth in trust, unbeknownst to his family, to fund the Nobel Prize awards. Nobel invented and made his fortune from dynamite. His wealth was estimated to be 31 million Swedish Kroner (SEK). Adjusted to the value of today's currency, this equates to approximately 1.794 billion SEK or over US$160 million. The Nobel Prize is not awarded posthumously.
154 Much along the lines of this book.
155 Monozygotic.
156 Dizygotic.

Some rare diseases, like sickle cell disease, Marfan's syndrome, and CADASIL[157], are caused by single gene mutations and can lead to strokes.[303,304]

Contrarian Thought
Could it be that we inherit the genes that control how our arteries are formed? And that we might be born with arteries that are more likely to develop atherosclerosis?

Contrarian Thought
Is it possible that more genes have not been found because we have been studying patients with **symptoms** of the disease atherosclerosis, not the **actual disease itself**? As already mentioned, this is looking at the tip of the iceberg.

Despite many hundreds of publications, results have been largely disappointing with few definite gene abnormalities identified.[305]

Contrarian (but not original) Thought
In the vast majority of us who suffer a stroke or heart attack, despite the fact that another member of our family may also have had a stroke or heart attack, it is likely that we have not inherited bad genes. We have, just like our relatives, grown older and developed worsening hardening of our arteries – unless my suggestion that we may inherit genes that mean our blood vessels form in a way that makes them more likely to develop atherosclerosis is correct.

---

157 Cerebral Autosomal Dominant Arteriopathy with Subcortical Infarcts and Leukoencephalopathy.

28. Cholesterol

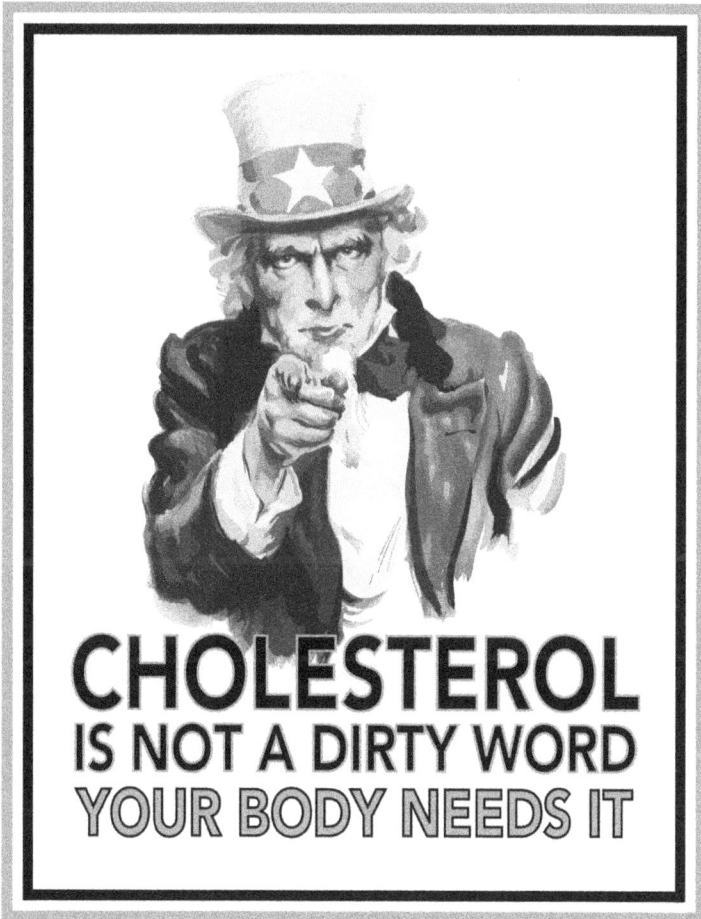

Figure 28.1. An adaptation of the US army advertising campaign created by James Montgomery Flagg in 1917, with Uncle Sam entreating citizens to enlist. It is simply stating that cholesterol is vital to our bodies. It is of course harmful when it accumulates in the walls of our arteries. This work is in the public domain in the United States because it was published (or registered with the US Copyright Office) before January 1, 1925.

Cholesterol is often seen as the enemy, with constant warnings in the media about its dangers and how we should lower it through diet, weight loss, or medication. Many people fear cholesterol because it is linked to heart attacks and strokes, as it builds up in our arteries. In fact, research on cholesterol has led to 13 Nobel Prizes.[306]

Why Cholesterol is Important

Despite its bad reputation, **cholesterol is essential for our bodies.** It is a type of fat that needs to combine with protein to move through our blood. Cholesterol with more protein is called high-density lipoprotein (HDL), or "good cholesterol," while cholesterol with less protein is called low-density lipoprotein (LDL), often called "bad cholesterol".

Our bodies cannot survive without cholesterol. Every cell makes a small amount, but most of it is produced in the liver through a complex process involving nearly 100 different genes.[307] LDL helps transport cholesterol from the liver to cells, while HDL recycles it back to the liver. Cholesterol is essential for:

- Building and repairing cells (our bodies replace billions of cells every day)[158].[57]
- Making bile salts, which help digest fat.
- Producing vitamin D and important hormones like cortisol, aldosterone, testosterone, oestrogen, and progesterone.
- Helping our bodies absorb vitamins A, D, E, and K.

Why Cholesterol Gets a Bad Name

Although cholesterol is crucial for health, it becomes a problem when it builds up in artery walls as we age. This increases the risk of heart attacks, strokes, and poor circulation to the legs.

Cholesterol in Food

Since early experiments showed that feeding cholesterol to rabbits caused droplets of lipid in the walls or their arteries, we've been told to avoid cholesterol-rich foods. However, our liver produces much more cholesterol than we get from our diet. When we eat more cholesterol, our livers usually produce less to balance it out. Only about 25% of people, called "hyper-responders," experience a small cholesterol increase from their diet.[308,309] Even in these people, the rise is usually only 10–15%[159].[308-310]

What is a Normal Cholesterol Level?

There is no universal agreement on what a normal cholesterol level is, and guidelines often change[160]. Generally, recommendations suggest lowering cholesterol, especially LDL.

---

158 It is estimated that we have a "new body" every 80 days.
159 Therefore, if the cholesterol is 5 mmol/L (193 mg/dL), it will only increase to 5.5–5.75 mmol/L (212–222 mg/dL) at most.
160 The current guidelines from the US, Europe and Britian are in Appendix E.

Familial Hypercholesterolaemia (FH)

Familial hypercholesterolaemia (a genetic condition caused by a mutation on chromosome 19) is rare; it occurs in less than 1% of the population. It results in very high LDL cholesterol from birth. People with one abnormal gene[161] have twice the normal cholesterol level[162], while those with two abnormal genes[163] (a rare condition) have levels four times higher[164]. FH leads to early heart disease, with symptoms appearing as young as 27 in men and 33 in women.[311] If untreated, those with two abnormal genes often die before 30 years of age. In 1938, the Norwegian scientist Dr Carl Müller recognised the link between elevated serum cholesterol levels, tendon xanthomas (fatty deposits), and the lesions in coronary arteries in patients with FH.[312]

However, varying rates of ASCVD events have been observed in patients with FH, even among individuals with identical genetic mutations and comparable LDL levels. Hence, other things that change ASCVD risk apart from LDL must contribute to the elevated ASCVD risk in the FH population.[313] Increasing age impacts risk in heterozygotes (people with one abnormal gene), just as it does in the broader population.[311]

If the evidence indicates that physical damage starts the process, this poses a question about what other factors contribute to premature development of atherosclerosis in patients with FH. The abnormal genes impair the uptake of LDL by the cells. When this affects the endothelial cells lining the arteries it causes them to not function normally. These cells become less flexible and more brittle. They no longer act like Teflon and this exposes the walls of arteries to more damage. One hypothesis is that the cells lining the inner wall of the arteries, the intima (the Teflon layer), are not as good at absorbing cholesterol, making this layer less flexible and more brittle – and therefore more susceptible to damage.[314] Impaired endothelial function has been documented in children with FH,[315,316] including changes that prevent their arteries from expanding enough to cope with the increased blood flow with each heartbeat. This dysfunction almost certainly makes it more likely that the arterial wall will be progressively damaged, allowing more cholesterol to seep into the artery wall.

When Should We Get Tested for FH?

Children should be tested if a parent has FH or has had a heart attack or stroke before the age of 50 without other major risk factors like obesity, diabetes, high blood pressure, or smoking.

People should also get tested if they develop yellowish cholesterol deposits (xanthomas) on their skin, especially around joints and tendons. Early treatment is critical to reduce risk, particularly in people with two abnormal genes.

---

161 Called heterozygotes.
162 350–550 mg/dL: 09.05–14.2 mmol/L.
163 Called homozygotes.
164 As high as 650–1,000 mg/dL (16.8–25.9 mmol/L).

Cholesterol, Heart Attack and Stroke Risk

Atherosclerosis (artery hardening) affects everyone to some degree, but not everyone experiences heart attacks or strokes.[317–320] High cholesterol is a known risk factor, but early studies found it had a clearer link to heart attacks than strokes. This is because strokes can have different causes, not all related to cholesterol build up in the arteries (atherosclerosis).

A 2022 analysis of many studies[165,166] found that people with the highest LDL levels had a slightly lower risk of strokes caused by burst blood vessels but an 11% higher risk of strokes caused by blocked arteries.[321] Very low LDL levels, less than 70 mg/dL (1.81 mmol/L) may increase the risk of brain bleeds,[322–325] though studies on cholesterol-lowering drugs haven't confirmed this risk.[326]

Important Takeaways

- Not everyone with high cholesterol develops heart disease or stroke, and not everyone with normal cholesterol is safe from heart disease or stroke.
- If we have obesity with high blood pressure, diabetes and particularly if we smoke, we cannot be reassured that we will be spared from a heart attack or stroke just because our cholesterol is normal.
- Focusing too much on cholesterol can distract us from other important risk factors like obesity and smoking.
- A high cholesterol level is one risk factor we can control. While the increased risk (ARI)$_{167}$ and the benefit (ARR)$_{11}$ of lowering cholesterol with drugs for an individual may seem small, this increased and decreased risk affecting millions of people worldwide translates to both a huge increase and decrease of the number of strokes and heart attacks.$_{11}$ Estimates suggest that in the US, 86 million adults over the age of 20 have elevated cholesterol.$_{168}$ The RRR$_{11}$ means there would be far fewer heart attacks and strokes if everyone had their high cholesterol treated.

---

165 A meta-analysis is a research process used to systematically synthesise or merge the findings of single, independent studies, using statistical methods to calculate an overall or 'absolute' effect. Egger, M., et al. (1998). "Meta-analysis Spurious precision? Meta-analysis of observational studies." BMJ 1998: 316(7125): 140–151.

166 The analysis undertaken by the Lipid and Blood Pressure Meta-Analysis Collaboration (LBPMC) Group and the International Lipid Expert Panel (ILEP). It involved 355,591 patients in observational studies and 165,988 patients in randomised controlled trials.

167 The ARI (absolute risk increase) and RRI (relative risk increase) represent the increased risk to the individual vs the increased risk of the whole population, whilst the ARR (absolute risk reduction) and RRR (relative risk reduction) represent the benefit to the individual vs the entire society respectively.

168 Centre for Disease Control and Prevention https://www.cdc.gov/cholesterol/data-research/facts-stats/?CDC_AAref_Val=https://www.cdc.gov/cholesterol/facts.htm.

How to Lower Cholesterol with Diet

Since we can't know if we are hyper-responders to dietary cholesterol, it's best to follow a heart-healthy diet. Harvard[169] Health[170] recommends eating:

- Whole grains like oats and barley
- Beans, eggplant, and okra
- Nuts (about 57g or 2oz per day)
- Vegetable oils
- Fruits like apples, grapes, strawberries, and citrus
- Foods with added sterols and stanols (found in some margarines, granola bars, and orange juice)
- Soy products like soy milk and tofu (25g per day)
- Fatty fish (2–3 times per week)[171]
- Fibre supplements like psyllium (found in Metamucil).

Note the lack of highly refined carbohydrates on this list. By making these dietary changes and managing other risk factors, chances of heart attack and stroke are reduced.

---

169 Harvard University is a private, highly respected Ivy League research university in Cambridge, Massachusetts, US.

170 https://www.health.harvard.edu/heart-health/11-foods-that-lower-cholesterol.

171 in reality there is not enough fish left in the oceans for everyone to have 2–3 serves per week. A 2012 BBC report pointed out that around 85% of global fish stocks are over-exploited, depleted, fully exploited or in recovery from exploitation with global fish consumption at 17kg (37lb) per year.

29. Diabetes

A Little History of Diabetes

The word "diabetes"[172] comes from a Greek word meaning "to siphon" because people with diabetes were known to pass large amounts of urine. There may be a reference to diabetes in an ancient Egyptian text[173] from 1500 BC.[327] In India, a 6th-century physician named Sushruta called it "Madhumeha," meaning "sweet urine," as people noticed that ants were attracted to the urine of those with diabetes. Sushruta suggested that diabetes was linked to being overweight and inactive.[328] This is still the case today. In the past, doctors would even taste urine to check for sweetness, but today we use test strips to detect diabetes.

The word "diabetes" first appeared in English medical texts around 1425. In 1675, Thomas Willis added the term "mellitus," meaning "honey-sweet," because of the sugar in the urine. Many ancient cultures, including the Greeks, Chinese, Egyptians, Indians, and Persians, had already noticed this.

In 1921, Frederick Banting and John Macleod discovered insulin, which helps control blood sugar by moving it into the cells for energy. Banting and Macleod were awarded the 1923 Nobel Prize. The first insulin injection was given at the Toronto General Hospital in Canada to 14-year-old Leonard Thompson in 1922. Later, scientists created artificial insulin using DNA technology.[329]

What is Diabetes?

Diabetes is a long-term condition where blood sugar levels are too high. People with diabetes can develop damage to the heart, blood vessels, eyes, kidneys, and nerves over time. The most common (90–95%) type is type 2 diabetes[174], which occurs when the body becomes resistant to insulin or doesn't make enough of it. This is usually linked to obesity. Type 1 diabetes, on the other hand, is an autoimmune disease where the body attacks insulin-producing cells[175] in the pancreas.

While insulin and medications can help control blood sugar, diabetes can continue causing damage without obvious symptoms until it is too late. It is often called the 'silent killer', with increased risk of kidney failure, heart attack, stroke, loss of sensation in the feet[176], increased tendency to develop infections and blindness.

---

172 A detailed account of the discovery of diabetes can be found on the following website: http://www.ncbi.nlm.nih.gov/pubmed/11953758 and in a wonderful paper by Marianna Karamanou and colleagues from the Department of History of Medicine, Medical School, University of Athens titled: Milestones in the history of diabetes mellitus: The main contributors. World J Diabetes. 2016 Jan 10;7(1): 1–7. https://doi.org/10.4239/wjd.v7.i1.1
173 The Eber's papyrus.
174 Also called type 2 diabetes.
175 It is not known what triggers the body to attack the islet cells in the pancreas. No single gene has been identified but a number of genes increase the chances of developing diabetes.
176 Peripheral neuropathy.

Can We Prevent Diabetes?

Type 1 diabetes cannot be prevented. However, type 2 diabetes can often be avoided by maintaining a healthy weight and staying active. Losing weight can prevent many people with prediabetes from developing full-blown diabetes.[330,331]

Prediabetes vs Diabetes

Prediabetes is when blood sugar levels are higher than normal but not high enough to be diagnosed as diabetes[177]. The cut-off point between prediabetes and diabetes is based on medical guidelines[178], but there isn't a perfect test for diagnosing diabetes. Blood tests are used to measure sugar levels, and an HbA1c test can show average blood sugar levels over the past few months.

HbA1c was discovered in 1968 by Samuel Rahbar in Iran[332]. It measures glucose attached to red blood cells. If the HbA1c level is above 6.5%, it indicates diabetes[179]. However, there is some debate about how best to diagnose and manage diabetes[180].[333]

Gestational Diabetes

Gestational Diabetes is a type of diabetes that occurs in women during pregnancy and usually disappears after the birth. However, women who have had gestational diabetes are at higher risk of developing type 2 diabetes later in life.

Symptoms and Risks

Many people with diabetes don't show symptoms at first, so testing is important, especially for people with excess weight. In the US, women with severe obesity (BMI>35kg/m^2) are up to an astonishing 93 times more likely to develop diabetes.[334] Symptoms of high blood sugar [180–200 mg/dL (10–11.1 mmol/L)] include blurry vision, excessive thirst, frequent urination, and fatigue.

177 National Institute of Diabetes and Digestive and Kidney Diseases https://www.niddk.nih.gov/health-information/diabetes/overview/what-is-diabetes/prediabetes-insulin-resistance.
178 Current guidelines based on a fasting blood glucose, tested twice, define prediabetes when the glucose is 100–125 mg/dL (5.3–6.9 mmol/L) and diabetes when the glucose is ≥126 mg/dL (7.0 mmol/L).
179 The Australian Pharmaceutical Benefits Scheme requires a HbA1c of >7% to approve use of the very expensive sodium glucose cotransporter-2 inhibitor (SGLT2i) and glucagon-like peptide-1 receptor agonist (GLP-1RA) drugs. Schedule of Pharmaceutical Benefits. Summary of Changes. Effective 1\u00a0April 2015. 2015. (accessed 12\u00a0March 2015.
180 The American College of Physicians (ACP) recommends less stringent goals as there are, in their opinion, harms associated with overzealous or inappropriate treatment focused on HbA1c targets. The ACP suggests we aim for an HbA1c in the range of 7–8%.

Type 1 diabetes symptoms can appear suddenly and be life-threatening. Without insulin, the body burns fat for energy, producing chemicals called ketones. Too many ketones can cause diabetic ketoacidosis (DKA), leading to nausea, vomiting, confusion, and coma. In type 2 diabetes, extreme high blood sugar[181] can also lead to a dangerous condition called hyperosmolar coma without excess ketones.

Diabetes, Heart Disease and Stroke

Diabetes doubles the risk of heart attacks and strokes.[335,336] The risk of stroke is tripled in patients who have diabetes for more than 10 years.[337] Scientists are still studying exactly how diabetes damages blood vessels. Postmortem studies of young patients and children with type 1 diabetes show more severe early changes of atherosclerosis (fatty streaks), even when cholesterol is not increased.[338,339] Blood sugar may damage the endothelial cells (Teflon-like lining) that protect the walls of arteries.[340–343]

Silent Heart Attacks

Somewhere between 12–35% of heart attacks may cause nausea, breathlessness, sweating, and fatigue but no chest pain, and these are called silent heart attacks[182]. People with diabetes are more likely to have heart attacks without the usual chest pain.[344,345]

Treating Diabetes

Managing diabetes requires controlling blood sugar levels[183] through diet, exercise, and medication.[292] Dietary advice can be found on American Diabetes Association,[12] the Diabetes Australia[184] and the European Association for the Study of Diabetes[346] (EASD)[185] websites. In the past, doctors noticed that diabetes improved when people lost weight. Food shortages during the Franco-Prussian War[328] and during World War II in Japan[347] and the Netherlands[186][348] led to fewer cases of diabetes. In the 1870s, Apollinaire Bouchardat a French pharmacist at the Hôtel-Dieu de Paris (a public hospital, despite the name), recommended increased exercise and a low-carb diet with more meat, cheese, eggs, and exercise – ideas that would be still useful today. Bouchardat also recognised how difficult it is to maintain weight loss with dieting[187].

---

181 Glucose levels can exceed 1,000 mg/dL (55.6 mmol/L), more than 150 times normal.
182 The medical term is silent myocardial ischaemia: myocardial means the heart muscle, and ischaemia is lack of oxygen. Lack of oxygen to our heart muscles causes a heart attack.
183 Recommended treatment can be found in the consensus report by the American Diabetes Association (ADA) https://diabetes.org/food-nutrition/food-and-diabetes.
184 Diabetes Australia website https://www.diabetesaustralia.com.au/living-with-diabetes/healthy-eating/.
185 https://link.springer.com/article/10.1007/s00125-023-.
186 The number of outpatient consultations at the Public Health Service of Amsterdam for newly diagnosed diabetes declined from 140 to two during the second half of the war, but by 1949 it was up to 212.
187 Bouchardat wrote: "it is difficult to refrain, and to continue thus, when man so much hungers after bread. Despite the most careful monitoring, despite the assurances of these unfortunates, it is true that this food will become fatal for them, since nothing averts them from it. A little later, tired of this treatment that does not end and exhausted, more morally than physically, the diabetics resume their starchy meals; the accidents reappear....and death arrives."

New research suggests that weight loss, especially over 15 kg, can help some people achieve long-term remission (more than 10 years) of type 2 diabetes. Weight loss surgery[349,350] and very low-calorie diets[351–355] have been successful in some cases. **Remission of type 2 diabetes with diet is now considered a realistic treatment goal.**[356]

Does Treating Diabetes Prevent Heart Disease?

Lowering blood sugar helps prevent small blood vessel damage in the eyes, kidneys, and nerves. However, research is still unclear about whether controlling blood sugar alone prevents heart attacks and strokes.[357] As type 2 diabetes is due to obesity, with the complications of high blood pressure and high cholesterol, managing these risk factors is important for overall health.

Final Thoughts

Diabetes is a serious condition, but type 2 diabetes can be prevented by maintaining a healthy weight and lifestyle. Ongoing research continues to improve treatment options, but staying active, eating well, and most importantly weight control can prevent or reverse diabetes in people who have gained excess weight, causing the diabetes.

30 Obesity

In the past mankind hunted and killed his food
now excess highly processed food hunts and kills mankind.

Obesity is a massive topic, and what is presented here is a brief summary. In late 2018 I typed the word obesity into Pubmed, the program on the internet doctors and researchers use to find references. It produced 294,727; four years later the number had increased to 427,674! In 2023, typing the word obesity into Google yields a mind-numbing 778,000,000 hits!

No book on stroke would be complete without discussing obesity as it is one of the most significant factors that increases our risk of stroke (and heart attack) at a younger age, leading to premature disability and death. Studies of genes using the technique known as genome-wide association studies have identified many genetic variants associated with obesity, but **they have not definitely proven that obesity is a genetic(inherited) disease.**[358–361]

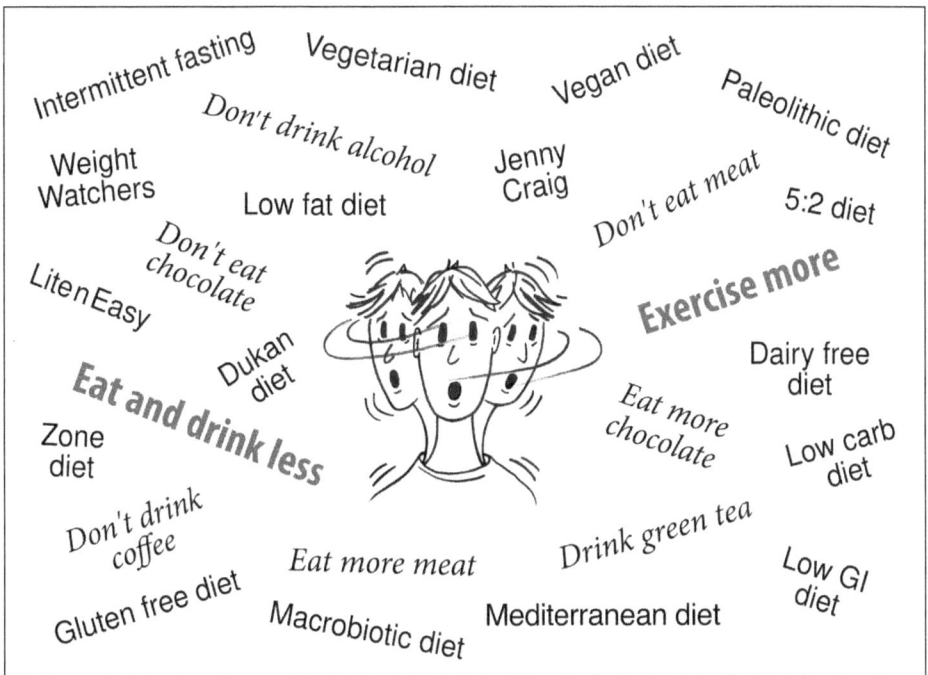

Figure 30.1 The bewildering world of obesity. Illustration Sandra Coventry.

The Bewildering World of Obesity

The world of obesity, as illustrated in Figure 30.1 is bewildering. Every day we are bombarded by conflicting lifestyle advice about what to and what not to eat and drink. The food, beverage, and weight loss industries are multibillion-dollar businesses with significant vested interests.

There is a vast amount of research sponsored by the food and beverage industry. It is rare for an industry-funded study to find something detrimental to that industry. On the contrary, they often claim benefit when other studies, not funded by industry, find exactly the opposite.[362] It is alleged that industry-funded research into sugar-sweetened beverages is 57 times, *yes 57 times* more likely than independently funded research to show results that are favourable to their products.[363] The proportion of studies of treatment with unfavourable conclusions was 0% for industry-funded research versus 37% for non-industry-funded research.[364]

Often it is impossible for us to know whether the studies are funded by industry as they frequently do not declare a potential conflict of interest. Their publication in scientific medical journals gives them legitimacy.[365] Any criticism of the food or beverage industry is immediately attacked in an attempt to discredit the research or the author. This is understandable; after all the food and beverage industry does not want us to consume less and be healthier as this would impact on their profits.

The field of dietetics and nutritional research is bedevilled by association studies and as we have made clear in a prior chapter association does not prove causation. Association studies are responsible for much of the confusion depicted in Figure 30.1. While very few scientists are accused of misconduct or misreporting data, critics have long contended that nutrition research is plagued by a credibility problem.[366–371] They argue that an alarming number of food studies are misleading, unscientific, or draw dubious conclusions.

We have elite sports people and movie stars recommending all sorts of fad diets, dietary supplements and it is doubtful that they have carefully researched the proof that what they are recommending to their fans is of proven value.[188] There is no evidence whatsoever to back up most of the claims of many of the trendy health products and practices endorsed by celebrities.[372]

There are literally thousands of websites that offer advice for healthy living. Very few of these websites quote the scientific basis for their claims. Some lifestyle gurus simply report the results of scientific studies without any critical appraisal of the validity of the study. Others try to entice us to buy their miraculous weight loss method and even offer us a money-back guarantee on their sure-fire way to rapidly lose weight if it does not work. The problems with the (mis) information on the internet are highlighted in the book "The Death of Expertise: The campaign against established knowledge and why it matters.[189]"[373]

---

188 It is my belief that they have a moral obligation to only recommend what is of proven value.
189 Well worth reading.

Fat Cell Numbers and Size

In childhood and adolescence weight gain is associated with an increased number and size of fat cells, referred to as hyperplastic[190] obesity. In adults weight gain is largely the result of increased fat in each fat cell, referred to as hypertrophic[191] obesity. Whether the number of cells increases in adulthood is uncertain as there is conflicting evidence.[374,375] It is estimated that the average person has roughly 30 billion fat cells.[376] When we lose weight the number of fat cells does not change. Like all cells, fat cells do not live forever; approximately 10% are turned over each year.

Warning the pictures on the following page
may offend some people.

They show 10kg bags of fat and how much fat we are carrying if we are 10, 20, 30 and 40 kg overweight.

---

190 The enlargement of tissue caused by an increase in the reproduction rate of its cells.
191 The enlargement of tissue from the increase in size of its cells.

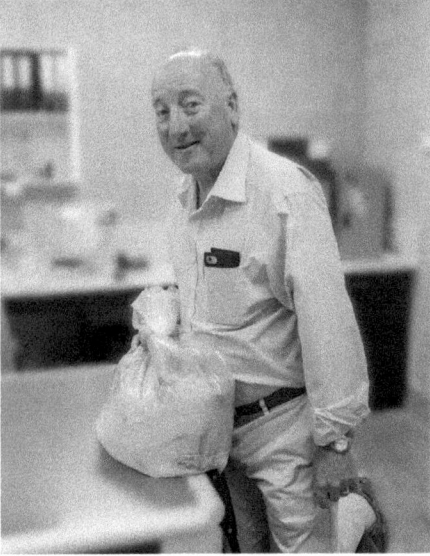

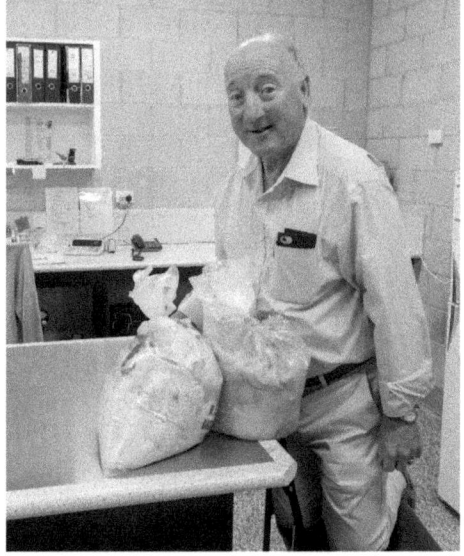

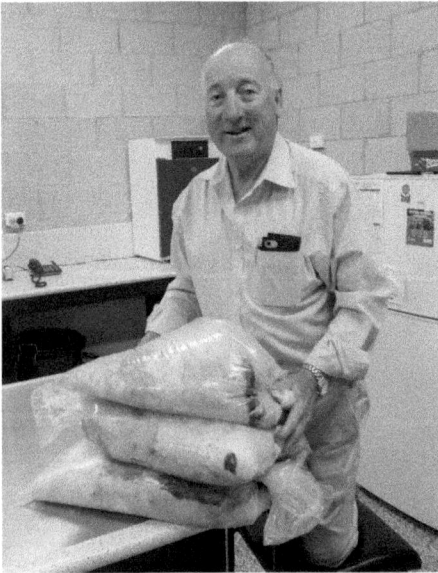

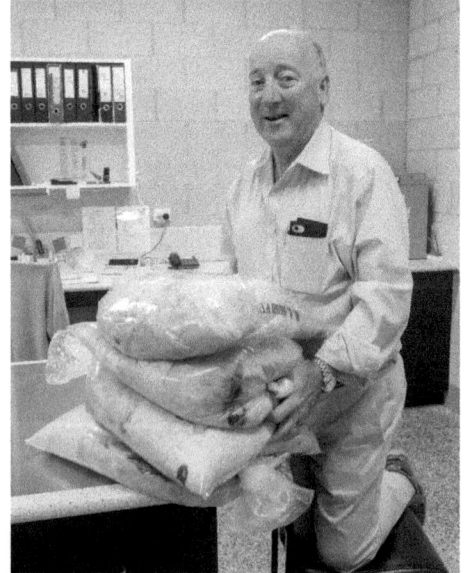

Figure 30.2a These images show 10kg bags of fat and how much fat we are carrying if we are 10, 20, 30 and 40kg overweight.

Bad Genes

A tiny number of us may inherit a "bad gene" from our parents that will cause obesity that is beyond our control. These are referred to as monogenic (due to a single gene abnormality) obesity disorders.[377] Monogenic obesity commences in early childhood, often in the first few months of life[378–385] and results in very severe obesity due to overeating. This is due to a mutation in the pathway[192] that controls our eating behaviour.

One of these monogenic disorders is Leptin deficiency.[386–388] These patients lose weight when given leptin.[193] When leptin was given to fat mice it made them thin but when it was given to obese individuals without leptin deficiency in the hope it might cause weight loss it failed miserably![389] Some lost weight, some gained weight and many had unacceptable side effects from the injection.

Several other single gene disorders have been reported[194] and it is likely that more will be discovered with the passage of time. To date, all the single gene forms of severe obesity are the result of increased appetite.[384]

The Prader-Willi syndrome[390] is where we inherit one gene from our mother and one from our father, but one is silenced or not working. This results in severe childhood obesity.[391] These unfortunate individuals are short, have intellectual disability, behavioural disturbances, difficulty walking and excessive hunger.

In most of us with obesity, no single genetic cause can be identified.[392] According to Sadia Saeed from Lille, France and many international co-authors on the paper, single gene disorders causing obesity is extremely rare and probably accounts for less than 5% of the obesity in our society.[393]

Excess Consumption and Obesity

A tiny proportion of us may have inherited an obesity gene, some may have a medical problem that can cause weight gain, such as low thyroid hormone (hypothyroidism), polycystic ovaries, or a tumour in our pituitary gland (situated inside our head just behind the bridge of our nose) just to mention a few. In one type of pituitary tumour weight gain is due to the secretion of excess cortisol. We also gain weight when we are prescribed cortisone to treat a medical problem. Drugs used to treat depression, psychosis, epilepsy, migraine, and diabetes can cause weight gain, as can the oral contraceptive.

---

192   leptin-melanocortin.

193   Leptin was discovered by Jeffrey Friedman at the Rockefeller in New York.

194   Recognised abnormal genes leading to obesity include: Leptin and leptin receptor deficiency, proopiomelanocortin (POMC) deficiency, Melanocortin Receptor 4 deficiency (MC4R), Prohormone convertase deficiency, brain-derived neurotrophic factor (BDNF) and its receptor, tropomycin receptor kinase B (TrkB) insufficiency, Single-minded 1 (SIM 1) insufficiency Syndromic obesity, Adipocyte-, C1q-, and collagen domain-containing (ADIPOQ), Peroxisome proliferator-activated receptor gamma (PPARG), Insulin-induced gene 2 (INSIG2), adenylate cyclase 3 (ADCY3), Prader–Willi syndrome, Bardet–Biedl syndromes, Beckwith–Wiedemann syndrome, Alstrom–Hallgren syndrome, Carpenter syndrome. This list is likely to expand over the ensuing years.

However, the reality is that in the **vast majority of us, obesity is the direct result of consuming more calories[195] than our body needs to function.** Our bodies store every ounce or gram of energy we consume, a throwback to the hunter-gatherer times when we wouldn't know when our next meal was coming.

Weight gain does not happen overnight; it sneaks up on us. It has been estimated that as little as a 120 calorie (500 kJ) daily positive balance, the equivalent of just one small chocolate bar would produce a 50kg increase in our weight over 10 years.[394]

Removing salt and fat from our diet (as recommended in the guidelines) means that the only food that tastes good is full of sugar! When John Yudkin wrote about the dangers of sugar in his book titled "Pure, White and Deadly"[73] he

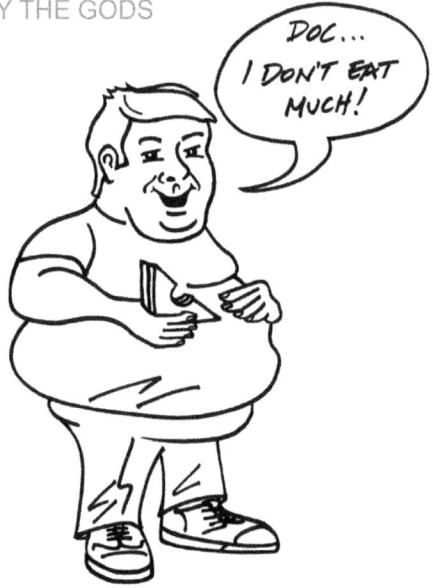

Figure 30.2b An illustration highlighting how little insight most of us have in terms of how much we eat. If we carry excess weight, we are eating too much. Illustration Sandra Coventry.

was pilloried, not only by the sugar industry but also by Ancel Keys the very man who published the flawed 7 Nations study. The critics of Yudkin correctly asserted that sugar is a natural substance and therefore it cannot be poison. It is not the sugar perse that is poisonous to our bodies but rather the massive amounts in the processed foods and the sugar-containing beverages we consume (Figure 30.3).

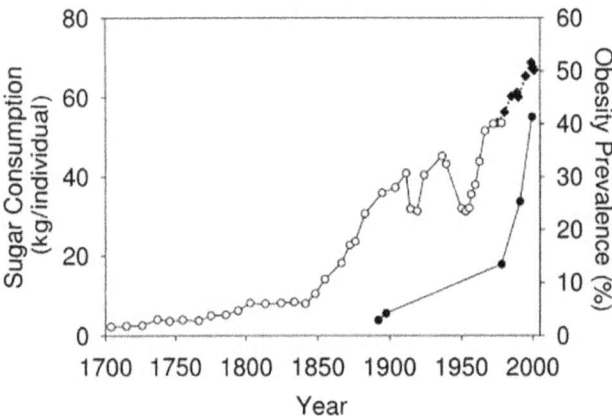

Figure 30.3: United Kingdom (open circles) and United States (dark squares) per person annual sugar consumption. (Source[395] who quotes Deer et al.[76] The line with the dark circles represents the increasing number of people with obesity.

---

195 Strictly speaking calories with a small c is 1000th of a Kilocalorie and when Calorie is written with a capital C this is a kilocalorie which is what most of us count when we count calories. In this book a lower-case c is used for both a calorie and a kilocalorie. It will be obvious from the context in which it is used as to what one is being discussed.

Yearly sugar consumption in the US and UK has increased from less than one kg per person in the 1700's up to almost 70kg per person in the year 2000. Sugar is often hidden in the food we purchase with at least 65 different names for sugar.[196]

We are consuming more sugar-sweetened beverages. In 1900 it was only 12 bottles per year per person. It peaked in 1999–2000 at 54 gallons (245 litres or 408, 600ml bottles). More than 50 countries have introduced taxes on sugar sweetened beverages,[197] with varying results. In 2016 Chile enacted laws that mandated front of package warnings, restricted child directed marketing and the banning of sales in schools of all foods and beverages containing added sugars, sodium or saturated fats that exceeded set nutrient and calorie thresholds. The result was a negligible 22.8 mL (0.77oz) per capita per day reduction in sugar sweetened beverage (SSB's) purchases.[396] A one peso (approximately five US cents) tax on SSB's decreased consumption by only 6%.[397] In 2015 in Germany, industry made voluntary commitments towards a national sugar reduction strategy. Six years later there was a negligible reduction in the sugar content of sugar sweetened beverages (2%) and sales of SSB's (4%).[398] In the United Kingdom on the other hand the introduction of a £0.24 per litre levy on SSB's containing more than 8 gm/100mL and a £0.18 per litre for those containing 5–8 gm/100mL had a significant impact. Industry reduced the sugar content of the highest SSB's but both increased the size (172mL) of their own-brand SSB's and the price of the SSB's with the higher levy. (£0.075/L)![399] No levy was placed on SSB's with < 5gm/100mL, fruit juice or pureed fruit without other added sugar, despite them having over 5gm/100mL of sugar. The levy resulted in a 43.7% (45 million kg) reduction in sugar content in sugar sweetened beverages and a massive 35.4% reduction in sugar consumption from sugar sweetened beverages. Unfortunately, there was an increased consumption of sugar sweetened beverages that were not taxed.[399,400]

It is not just excess sugar that is the problem. In the US where figures are readily available, meat (protein) consumption has more than doubled over the last century, by 2020 it was 264 lb. (120kg) per person, per year.[401] Carbohydrates consumption increased by approximately 25% between 1980 and 2000 and fat consumption increased by more than one-third between 1980 and 2010.[402] The number of calories we consume is up from 1,500 in the 1700s to 3,500 per day in the early 21st century (Figure 30.4).

The population in the United States increased from 90 million in 1900 to 314 million by 2012. US meat consumption increased from 10 billion lb. (4.53 billion kg) in 1909 to 55 billion lb (24.8 billion kg) in 2012. Thus, the population increased 3.5-fold whilst meat consumption increased 5.5-fold. The per capita consumption

---

196 The UK Health Science Academy. https://thehealthsciencesacademy.org/wp-content/uploads/2014/08/The-Health-Sciences-Academy_65-Names-Of-Sugar.pdf Sadly, Australia has yet to introduce a tax on sugar in sugar sweetened beverages.

197 a detailed report on the influence of taxes on sugar sweetened beverages can be found in the Obesity Evidence Hub. https://www.obesityevidencehub.org.au/collections/prevention/countries-that-have-implemented-taxes-on-sugar-sweetened-beverages-ssbs#:~:text=The%20UK%20tax%20led%20to,from%20soft%20drinks%20each%20year.

Daily supply of calories per person 1274 to 2022

Measured in kilocalories per person per day. This indicates the calories that are available for consumption, but does not necessarily measure the number of calories actually consumed, since it doesn't factor in consumer waste.

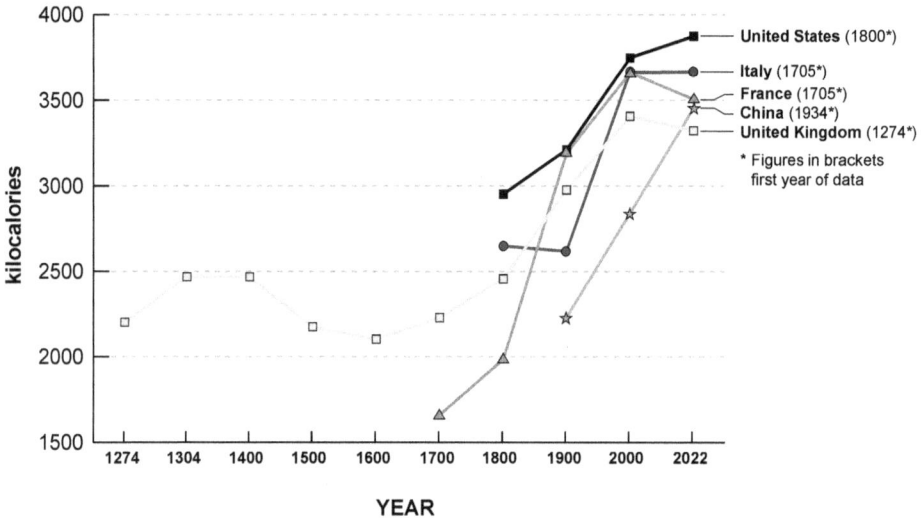

Figure 30.4 Per capita daily supply of calories 1274-2022. When physical activity is declining the US and UK have seen a 31% increase, whilst France has increased by 53%. China has increased by 35% in a little over 100 years.

has gone from 100 lb. (45.4kg) per year to 180 lbs. (81.6 kg) per year. Quoting US figures is not to single out the US; the obesity epidemic has spread like wildfire throughout the world. It is simply that reliable statistics are available for the US.

The evidence is crystal clear. The epidemic of obesity is being fed by overconsumption in the setting of an increasingly sedentary lifestyle.

How Much We Should Weigh

Excess weight can be measured in two ways, body mass index(BMI) and waist circumference to height ratio(WHR).

To measure our WHR we simply divide our height by the circumference of our waist measured one cm above our umbilicus (belly button). The ideal ratio is <0.5, so, our 1.70m tall man must have a waist circumference of <85 cm. This measurement recognises that it is the fat around the organs in our stomach that is the major threat to our health.

To calculate our BMI, we divide our weight in kilograms by our height in metres multiplied by itself. i.e., weight/(height*height). e.g., if we are 1.70m tall and weigh 95Kg our BMI is 95/(1.7*1.7) or 32.9Kg/m^2 placing us in the obese range.

A body mass index(BMI) of 25 is ideal as it predicts a longer and healthier life. To see what our weight should be we simply measure our height in metres and multiply our height by itself, and then multiply that figure by 25. e.g., if we are 1.7 m tall our ideal weight should be (1.7*1.7 = 2.89) *25. =72.3 Kg.

Why is Obesity Dangerous?

Obesity adds extra strain on the joints of our back and legs leading to pain and difficulty walking due to osteoarthritis.[403] Obesity increases the amount of blood our arteries have to pump around our body; this increases our blood pressure resulting in worsening physical damage to our arteries. There is an increase in the numbers and size of our fat cells, so our body has to increase its cholesterol production to help maintain these cells. The increased cholesterol in our blood causes more cholesterol to form on the inside of our arteries, resulting in atherosclerosis. If we are obese, our bodies cannot produce enough insulin, so our blood sugar rises and we develop type II diabetes. The high blood pressure, high cholesterol and diabetes that occur with obesity all increase our risk of heart attack and stroke.[404]

Life expectancy had increased from 41 years in Elizabethan times (late 16th century) to 54 just prior to the 1918 Spanish flu that killed 20% of its victims, mainly the young and healthy. As a result, life expectancy plummeted to 47 years. Since 1918 life expectancy has almost doubled to more than 80 years of age in many first world countries[198]. Figure 30.5 shows how many 40-year-old males would still be alive every 10 years between 50 and 100 years of age with a BMI

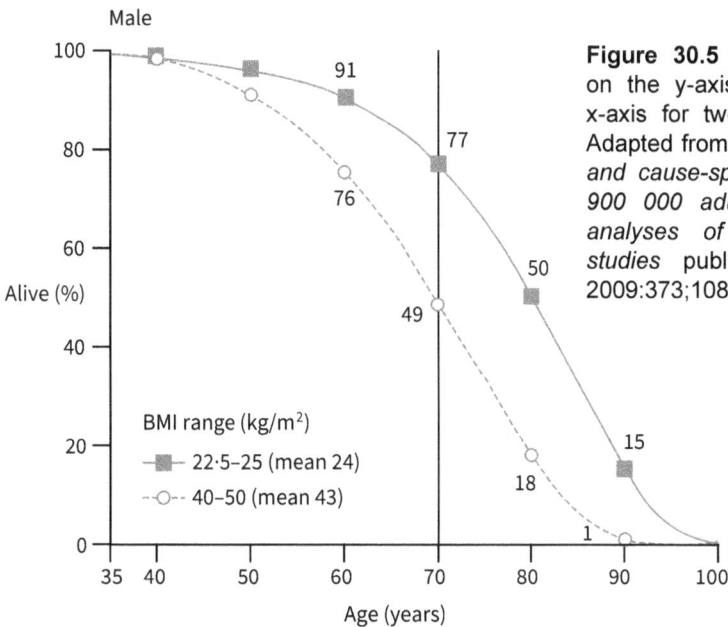

Figure 30.5 Plots % survival on the y-axis vs age on the x-axis for two different BMI's. Adapted from *Body-mass index and cause-specific mortality in 900 000 adults: collaborative analyses of 57 prospective studies* published in *Lancet* 2009:373;1083-1096.[406]

---

198 A wonderful discussion by Steven Johnson on the history of life expectancy can be found at: chrome-extension://efaidnbmnnnibpcajpcglclefindmkaj/https://pulitzercenter.org/sites/default/files/2021-04/05_02Longevity._NYTSHIPPED.pdf.

between 22.5 and 50 kg/m². At age 70, 77% of us with the lowest BMI will be still alive as opposed to only 49% with the highest BMI. Twenty-four per cent with the highest BMI will already be dead by the age of sixty! Only nine per cent of us with an ideal BMI of 25kg/m² will die before the age of 60. Morbid obesity (BMI ≥ 40 kg/m²) increases the death rate by a mind-boggling 30-fold compared to those with a BMI <25 kg/m².[405] Life expectancy is reduced by 8–10 years in patients with a BMI of 40–45kg/m².[406]

Calories in Calories Out

Our weight reflects the balance between the number of calories our body needs to function and how many we consume. How many we need depends on whether we are male or female, our age, how much we weigh and our level of physical activity. In essence, most adults between the ages of twenty and forty need 2400–3000/day. Our daily calorie needs diminish over the age of forty. Chapter 38 provides detailed tables that show how many calories we need, how many we burn up with different types of activity and how much exercise we need to do to burn all the calories in a hamburger, packet of potato crisps, bottle of soft drink or two scoops of ice-cream.

Counting calories is difficult; a straightforward way to see if we are consuming too many is to weigh ourselves on a regular basis, perhaps weekly. There will be some variation from day to day, but if we are gaining weight, we are consuming too many calories and need to cut back on how much we are eating, increase our level of physical activity, or preferably both. There are fewer calories to use for energy or to store as fat when we eat protein than when we eat fat and carbohydrate because it takes 25% more calories for our body to process protein. A not unreasonable approach is to count the calories we consume each meal for 1 week. Then we can see where we can cut back, simply by reducing the amount of food and beverages, we consume.

There are 3500 calories in 1kg of fat, if we reduce our consumption by 500 calories per day or increase our exercise, so we use an extra 500 calories per day, we could lose 1kg each week. If we do both, we could potentially lose 2kg/week. It really is that simple, but clearly, it is not that easy; otherwise, we would not have so many obese people in the world. It is very much like a colleague once said, "I don't know what the fuss is about giving up smoking; it is easy I have done it hundreds of times!" The same applies to obesity, many of us have lost weight only to regain it.

Our bodies do not want us to lose weight, a throwback to when food was scarce. When we try, our body releases a hormone that increases hunger and decreases the amount of the hormone that reduces hunger,[199] the effect of these two changes are to make us hungry. This together with the fact that we *live in an obesogenic environment* with an overabundance of appetite stimulating, addictive highly processed, high-calorie content, low fibre food and beverage in the setting of an increasingly sedentary lifestyle.

---

199 The hormone that increases appetite is called ghrelin, the hormone that decreases our hunger is called leptin.

Highly Processed Foods and Addiction

Highly processed foods, created to maximize flavour, "fool our brain" and coerce us to eat more calories than we would if presented with the same number of calories in unprocessed foods.[407] It has been suggested that highly processed food is as addictive as tobacco[408] and those processed foods with added sweeteners and fats, demonstrate the greatest addictive potential![409,410] The prevalence (proportion of the population) with food addiction is of the order of 20%.[411]

This would suggest highly processed foods are a major cause of the obesity epidemic, but as pointed out above the epidemic can be blamed on excess consumption of calories from carbohydrates, fat, protein, and sugar sweetened beverages in the setting of a more sedentary lifestyle.

If it is true that highly processed foods are addictive and entice us to eat more, then perhaps if we were to eat less highly processed foods it may be easier to eat less and lose weight, this is not easy. Gearhardt [412] has suggested that we may need to look to societal changes similar to those that were imposed to limit smoking – making cigarettes less affordable and less widely marketed – and do the same with addictive food. In 2009 the NOVA food processing classification system was proposed and has become the most prominent system in research and policy discussions.[413] The NOVA system groups foods into 1 of the following categories according to the extent and purpose of industrial processing:

- unprocessed,
- minimally processed foods,
- processed culinary ingredients,
- processed foods, and
- ultra-processed foods (UPF). NOVA specifically identifies foods that belong to the UPF category as problematic from a health perspective.

Although carbonated drinks have been shown to increase the hunger hormone ghrelin in rats,[414] there is no evidence in humans.

Our Body is like a Hybrid Car

Our bodies can be likened to a hybrid car. The hybrid car has two sources of fuel, electricity and when that runs out, petrol (gasoline). Our body has three sources of fuel. The primary one is glucose in carbohydrates. Whilst most of the cells of our body, particularly our brain use glucose, the cells of our heart and muscles, and the cells of our kidneys also use fatty acids, derived from fat to provide a substantial amount of their energy needs[200].

---

200   https://www.nature.com/scitable/topicpage/dynamic-adaptation-of-nutrient-utilization-in-humans-14232807/.

As long as we feed the cells of our body enough glucose, there is no need for them to switch to an alternative source of fuel, namely fat, the second main fuel source. The third source and one of last resort is protein. If we do not eat enough carbohydrate, once our bodies have used up the four gm of sugar (15 calories) floating around in our blood, they turn to the glucose we have stored as glycogen in our liver (400gm) and muscles (100gm)[201]. When our glycogen runs out, we switch to fat for energy. In severe starvation, once we deplete our fat stores, our body, as a last resort to survive, breaks down our muscles to keep us alive.

Burning fat produces ketones that our body uses for energy instead of glucose.[415] This is the "keto diet." Ketones prevent increased ghrelin secretion and thus suppress our appetite.[416] Ketones are the result of burning fat; thus, we will rapidly lose weight on a keto diet, as much as 18kg (40lb) in eight weeks.[417] On the other hand, if we replace the calories in carbohydrates with sufficient calories from fat to satisfy our bodies' energy needs, we will not lose weight.[418] The influence of excess protein on ketosis is less clear with claims that it does or does not reverse ketosis whilst on the keto diet with no scientific evidence provided to justify either of these claims. Currently a keto diet consists of roughly 55–60% fat, 30–35% protein and 5–10% carbohydrate (50gm of sugar). It is described as a quick fix diet for rapid weight loss that is hard to sustain in the long-term and once off it, we usually revert to our old eating habits and inevitably regain the weight, as we do with most diets.

There are supporters and opponents of the keto diet.[419] Proponents suggest that "the low-carbohydrate diet has failed and made the population sick." Opponents claim that there is no scientific proof of the superiority, safety, and sustainability of the ketogenic diet. In 2020 CNN published an article titled "experts say the keto diet isn't sustainable, so why is it so popular?"[202]. The article stated that these 24 experts ranked the keto diet almost last in the US News and World report on the 35 popular weight loss programs[203]. Experts are not always correct. Galen was an expert and he misled the world for centuries.

In reality, the process of ketosis is the normal way our body keeps us alive if we are deprived of carbohydrates.

---

201 A total of 2337 Calories is stored in glycogen.
202 https://edition.cnn.com/2020/01/05/health/keto-diet-day-wellness/index.html.
203 https://edition.cnn.com/2020/01/02/health/best-diet-worst-diet-2020-wellness/index.html.

A Cautionary Tale on Exogenous Ketones

There are claims on the internet and in the popular press that eating or drinking (exogenous) ketones can cause significant weight loss. "Keto Excel Keto Gummies[204] are easy-to-digest soft gel capsules that help lose weight, enhance mobility, flush out harmful chemicals and can achieve a healthy body with regular use." This sounds like the 21st centuries equivalent of 19th century snake oil.

However, when we look into it, we initially get the impression that there may be more to the use of exogenous ketones in weight loss. A review article states that drinking ketones reduce our appetite compared to sugar drinks.[416] This is the paper by Professor Stubbs discussed below. Exogenous ketones are reported to decrease our ghrelin level, thus suppressing our appetite.[420] If this results in us eating less, we will lose weight. Research suggests mice lose weight when fed ketones because they eat less, but one type, a synthetic, not natural ketone (R/S 1,3-Butanediol Acetoacetate Diester and 1,3-Butanediol) caused weight loss that was not accounted for by the mice eating less.[421]

The review by Deemer et al[416] is from a very respectable university and published in a highly respected journal. They quote a study that support the claims exogenous ketones suppresses appetite.[420] The paper quotes two other studies that failed to find any suppression of appetite.[422,423] Looking at the fine print in the positive study reveals that the author, Professor Kieran Clarke is a director of TDS Ltd., a company spun out of the University of Oxford to develop and commercialize products based on the science of ketone bodies in human nutrition. Clearly a potential conflict of interest that could lead to bias.

To complicate matters more, the "KetoExcel Gummies" touted on the internet contain extracts from irvingia gabonensis a fruit like a mango native to West Africa, an extract from the acai berry native to South America, the seeds of guarana a climbing plant native to the Amazon as well as other "natural substances" but NO ketones!

Food Pyramids

In 1943 the US Department of Food and Agriculture[205] published the "Basic 7" food guide, but the grouping made little sense. It was born out of hardship to help citizens to cope with the food rationing during the war.[206] The guide advised what should be eaten, largely based on the work of W.O. Atwater, Professor of Chemistry at Wesleyan College in Connecticut. Atwater published extensively on nutrition[424,425] and is considered the father of modern nutrition research and education. He founded

204 https://www.outlookindia.com/outlook-spotlight/keto-excel-keto-gummies-reviews-australia-nz-keto-excel-gummies-shocking-report-reveals-must-read--news-255451.
205 A detailed review of the evolution of the USDA dietary guidelines can be found in the Smithsonian Institute Magazine. https://www.smithsonianmag.com/smart-news/travel-back-time-these-old-usda-dietary-guidelines-180957741/#:~:text=1894%3A%20Farmer's%20Bulletin&text=The%20USDA%20first%20got%20into,be%20thought%20about%20and%20consumed.
206 The Freelance Star Fredericksburg, Va https://news.google.com/newspapers?id=qXNhAAAAIBAJ&pg=4981,1684677.

the first agricultural experimental station in the US and in his 1902 publication in the Farmers Bulletin [425] Atwater advocated variety, proportionality and moderation; measuring <u>calories</u>; and an efficient, affordable diet that focused on nutrient-rich foods and less fat, sugar and <u>starch</u>. It has all been said before.

The idea of using a pyramid to illustrate what to eat was the brainchild of Anna Britt Agnsäter, a home economics teacher who was the head of the test kitchen for Kooperativa Förbundets a Swedish consumers' cooperative federation. In 1974 Agnsäter simplified and visually clarified the confusing circular nutritional graphic which showed the elements that should be eaten and in which quantities and transformed it into the nutritional pyramid graphic that we know today.

Every country has its own recommendations designed to inform us about healthy eating. Many countries use the food pyramid. The Chinese use a pagoda, the Japanese a spinning top, the British an "eat-well" plate, the French food stairs, Australia has both a pyramid and a plate, and the Arabs have a food dome. They are all different, reflecting the types of food consumed in their own society. Italians are advised to eat pasta, bread, rice, olive oil, and salami, and drink wine in moderation. One litre of milk per day is recommended in Canada. Rice is recommended in China and Japan. The American food pyramid advises eating less rice and pasta!

Contrarian Thought

The pyramid in Figure 30.6 is one that would be of benefit to all societies regardless of the type of food and beverages they consume.

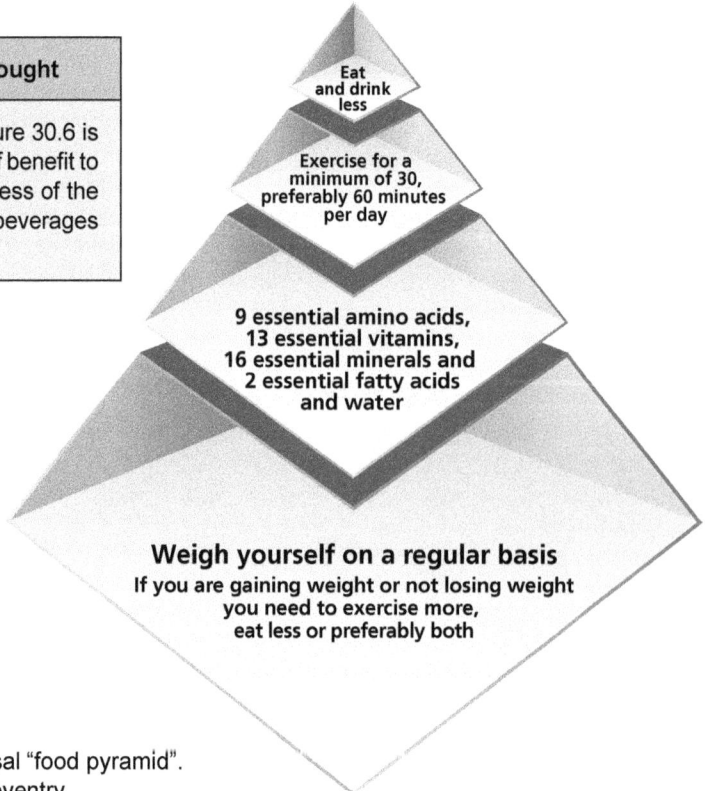

Eat and drink less

Exercise for a minimum of 30, preferably 60 minutes per day

9 essential amino acids, 13 essential vitamins, 16 essential minerals and 2 essential fatty acids and water

Weigh yourself on a regular basis
If you are gaining weight or not losing weight you need to exercise more, eat less or preferably both

Figure 30.6 A universal "food pyramid".
Illustration Sandra Coventry.

Eat Less Live Longer

In 1934 the life expectancy of rats was increased by a staggering 33% (four years instead of three) when they were fed far fewer calories.[426] Animal experiments with reduced calories have increased the life-expectancy of bacteria, worms, mice, and monkeys.[427] How many fat people do we see in their nineties and how many morbidly obese people do we see in their eighties or even seventies. The answer is few. Those of us who have long-lived parents often have a long life. We assume we have inherited a longevity gene. Indeed, many genes have been associated with longevity but only two consistently with repeated genome wide association studies.[428]

Throughout the entire animal kingdom, the secret to living a longer, healthier life is caloric restriction, i.e., not putting on excess weight![426,429] We have already described the Okinawan's and other long-lived societies. Those of us who remain lean throughout our entire lives are more likely to enjoy a healthier and longer life.[430]

There is one advantage of carrying excess fat; we will not starve to death as quickly. If we are lean, we will die after approximately 60 days (when we would lose more than 35% of our body weight) provided we drink water.[431] On the other hand Mr Angus Barbieri in Dundee Scotland, who weighed 456lb (207kg) survived starvation with no ill effects for an astonishing 382 days.[432]

Diets, Diets Everywhere

The illustration at the commencement of this chapter says it all. There is a bewildering number of different diets, it is no wonder we are confused. Should we go on a low-fat, high protein, keto, or Mediterranean diet? The Mediterranean diet is the one currently in favour and consists of little red meat, low to moderate amounts of fish, poultry, and large quantities of fruit, vegetables, whole grains, and…unrestricted olive oil as a source of monounsaturated fatty acids… however, simply adding olive oil to a diet that is already heavily supplemented with sugars and saturated fat, will end up adding more calories to an already high-calorie diet[207]."

In a review of the Mediterranean diet[433] the authors make the following statement. "The negative effects of obesity are partly reversed by substantial weight loss that can be achieved with the Mediterranean diet, especially if low-calorie and in combination with adequate physical activity." i.e., The Mediterranean diet is the same as all effective diets, they contain fewer calories than our bodies need and thus we have to start burning our fat deposits for energy. A 2016 review suggested that the Mediterranean diet results in similar weight loss in overweight and obese individuals trying to lose weight.[434] A comparison with the ketogenic diet showed both achieved significant weight loss and loss of body fat mass, the ketogenic diet was quicker.[435] Fewer calories is only one of the two features that all diets have in common. The other feature is that the weight we lose whilst dieting is most often regained because we return to our previous lifestyle that caused the obesity in the first place.

---

207   Attributed to Dr David Heber at UCLA.

Drugs and Surgery for Weight Loss

This is covered in Chapter 39. Drugs for weight loss are similar to diets. Weight is regained once they are stopped.

Summary

Essentially, removing salt and fat from our diet removed two of the three ingredients that make food tasty, leaving only sugar for taste. The food and beverage industry are making billions of dollars selling us appetite stimulating, addictive highly processed refined carbohydrates. The weight loss industry is making billions of dollars helping us with our life-long struggle to lose weight caused by the excess consumption of calories. The pharmaceutical industry is making billions of dollars selling us the drugs to treat the complications of obesity, namely, high blood pressure, diabetes and a high cholesterol. And now they have invented the "holy grail" drug[208], injections that suppress our appetite and help us to potentially lose massive amounts of weight. We need these injections for life, as the moment we stop them, we regain weight. I am now 10 kg lighter than I was at my heaviest, when my BMI was hovering at the obese level. I have done this by not dieting but changing my lifestyle. I have increased the amount of exercise I undertake and cut back on the amount of food I eat, with the occasional relapse. I intend to lose more.

Key Points
Our bodies extract and store as fat every ounce (gm) of energy it can from what we eat and drink. This is right down to the last two feet (0.6m) of our large bowel where fatty acids are extracted from the fibre we eat when it is broken down by the bacteria that live in our colon (large intestine). If we continue to consume more calories than our body needs, we will gain weight, it is that simple.
If we want to lose weight, we must eat and drink less calories and preferably exercise more. Nutritionists argue that it is not that straightforward, but every time I and my friends have lost weight (yes, I have had to battle the bulge) we did so by eating less and exercising more. Regaining the weight is even easier!
To avoid regaining the weight we lose, we need to adopt a "life-long" pattern of altered behaviour such that we do not consume more calories than our body needs to function.

---

208 The GLP1 receptor agonists.

31. High Blood Pressure

Other than not smoking and avoiding obesity, treating high blood pressure (hypertension) is one of the most important ways to prevent strokes.

Understanding Hypertension

Hypertension is the medical term for high blood pressure. Blood pressure (BP) is measured using a cuff that inflates around our arm, which momentarily blocks the blood flow in the artery. It records two numbers:

- Systolic (the first number) is when blood flow can be detected in the artery as the cuff is deflated, and a knocking sound is heard.
- Diastolic (the second number) is when the knocking sound is no longer heard as the cuff is deflated further.

A normal blood pressure is around 120–130/80, while high blood pressure is defined as above 140/90 (130/80 in the US).

A History of Blood Pressure Measurement

Doctors first started studying blood pressure in the 1700s[209].[436] In one early experiment, an English scientist named Reverend Stephen Hales inserted a glass tube attached to a brass pipe into a horse's artery and saw the blood rise over 8 feet in the tube! Over time, doctors developed safer ways to measure blood pressure. The first inflatable cuff, similar to the ones used today, was invented in the 19th century by the Austrian physician Samuel Siegfried Karl Ritter von Basch. The French physician Jean Poiseuille invented the mercury manometer (pressure gauge) to measure blood pressure. The instrument our doctors use to listen to our hearts and chests is the stethoscope[210]. It was invented in the early 19th century by Frenchman Renè Laennec. The idea came to him when he had difficulty hearing the breath sounds in a very obese patient using the traditional 19th century method of placing his ear up against the chest wall. He rolled paper into a cylinder and applied one end to his ear and the other to the chest. Finding that this helped him hear the breath sounds more clearly, from there he invented the stethoscope.[437] Modern technology has done away with the need for a stethoscope to measure blood pressure; it is all done electronically with a cuff around the arm.

---

209 A more detailed and fascinating history of the evolution of measuring blood pressure was presented to the Royal Society of Medicine in 1977 by Dr Jeremy Booth.
210 From Greek , stéthos – chest and σκοπή, skopé – examination.

What is a Normal Blood Pressure?

In 1975, when I finished medical school, doctors considered normal blood pressure to be 100 plus a person's age. Over time, research has shown that lower blood pressure reduces the risk of heart disease and strokes, so the definition of normal blood pressure has changed. An ideal blood pressure is 130–140/80–90, the lower figure is that recommended in the US.

Why is High Blood Pressure Dangerous?

Doctors didn't fully understand how dangerous high blood pressure was until the 20th century. It was the famous Framingham study that showed that people with very high blood pressure (>160/95) were four times more likely to have a stroke. [438]

The 1988 Veterans Administration study showed the benefits of treating severe (diastolic levels of 115–129mmHg) hypertension[211].[439] There was an astonishing 83% relative risk reduction (RRR) and a 36% absolute risk reduction (ARR), with numbers needed to treat (NNT) of only 3.3. There were 4 deaths in the patients given a placebo compared with none in the treated group. No heart attacks, no heart failure, and only 1 stroke occurred in those treated compared to 2 heart attacks, 1 stroke, 1 TIA, and 2 with heart failure in the placebo group. Damage to the blood vessels in the eyes occurred in 11 untreated patients and none in the treated group.

Today, the World Health Organization (WHO)[271] and European health authorities[270] recommend treatment if blood pressure is above 140/90 mmHg. In the United States, guidelines are stricter, with treatment recommended if blood pressure is 130/80 mmHg or higher.[272]

These changes are based on studies showing that lowering blood pressure reduces the risk of stroke and heart attack. Research like the PROGRESS and SPRINT trials provided strong evidence that treating high blood pressure more aggressively leads to better health outcomes (fewer strokes and heart attacks).[440,441]

Does Hypertension Cause Symptoms?

Most of the time, high blood pressure doesn't cause symptoms. Some people only find out they have it when the doctor measures their blood pressure during a visit. However, extremely high blood pressure (above 220/120) can cause blurred vision, confusion, drowsiness, chest pain, and nausea.

---

211 There was an astonishing 83% relative risk reduction (RRR) and a 36% absolute risk reduction (ARR), with numbers needed to treat (NNT) of only 3.3.

What Causes High Blood Pressure?

The exact cause of hypertension in most people is said to be unknown. This is called essential[212] hypertension. It is more common in people who are overweight. Appendix B[213] contains my published paper, which indicates that atherosclerosis with stiffening of our arteries and excess blood in our arteries related to obesity are the cause, simply because these occur decades before we develop high blood pressure.

Rarely, high blood pressure is caused by another medical condition, such as kidney disease or hormone imbalances. This is called secondary hypertension[214].

How Does Hypertension Cause Strokes?

High blood pressure can cause strokes in two ways:

1. Bleeding stroke: When blood pressure is too high, a blood vessel can burst, causing bleeding in the brain.
2. Blocked artery stroke: High blood pressure damages arteries, making it easier for clots to form and block blood flow.

Populations Without Hypertension

Some people groups never develop high blood pressure. A 1929 study found that in a Kenyan community, no one had a blood pressure above 126/86, and there were no cases of heart disease or stroke.[81] In 1929 the average blood pressure of a 60-year-old European was 140/90. In the Amazon's Yanomami tribe, where people eat very little salt and stay thin throughout life,[442] their blood pressure was an amazing 95/61 mmHg. Other societies, such as the Xingu of Brazil and the natives of Papua New Guinea and Kenya all have BMIs of 20–23 kg/m^2 – and do not have hypertension.[442]

Salt and Blood Pressure

Eating too much salt can raise blood pressure.[443,444] Most of us are eating a little more than 10 gm of salt per day,[445] far more than the current recommendation of less than 5 gm.[215] [446,447] More than 70% of the salt we consume comes from packaged, processed, and restaurant foods,[448] not from adding salt at the table. The biggest sources of hidden salt are bread, processed meats, sauces, and

---

212 The word essential implies the cause is unknown.
213 www.understandingneurology.com.au.
214 Secondary causes include renal artery stenosis (narrowing of the artery to the kidney) and kidney damage from various diseases; excess adrenaline and/or noradrenaline from a tumour (called a pheochromocytoma) in the adrenal gland, a small gland on top of our kidney; Cushing's syndrome with excess cortisone produced by a tumour in either our adrenal gland or our pituitary gland (a gland inside our head above and behind the bridge of our nose that secretes many hormones to control various functions of our body); and excess cortisone prescribed by doctors.
215 https://www.who.int/data/gho/indicator-metadata-registry/imr-details/3082.

spreads. Fast food meals can contain nearly 90% of the recommended daily salt intake, and a single hamburger contains a little over 1 gm.[449]

Soft (soda) drinks, particularly diet soft drinks [450] contribute to excess salt in our diet, if we have too many of them. The average consumption in the US is eight 355 ml (12oz) cans or bottles per week.

Even though health experts recommend reducing salt intake, the amount of sodium in packaged foods is not decreasing.[451]

Studies show that by reducing our salt intake by 6 mg/day, we can lower our systolic blood pressure by nearly 6 mmHg.[452]

Obesity and Blood Pressure

There is a strong link between being overweight and having high blood pressure, even in children.[453–455] Forty-five percent of us with a BMI of 18.5–24.9 will have high blood pressure, whilst high blood pressure occurs in 87% of us with morbid obesity (BMI more than 40 kg/m²).[456] Losing weight can significantly reduce blood pressure. During World War II, when food was scarce, people in West Germany and Finland lost weight, and their blood pressure dropped. An 8 kg loss can lower our BP by 14/13 mm Hg. It can also reverse enlargement of the heart caused by hypertension.[457]

Why Lowering Blood Pressure Matters

Many studies have confirmed the reduced risk of heart attack and stroke with treatment of high blood pressure.[458–463] Lowering systolic blood pressure by as little as 10 mmHg can reduce the risk of heart disease and stroke by 20%[216], a significant benefit to the overall population.[464]

Conclusion

- High blood pressure is not inevitable – some populations never develop it.
- Obesity, and to a lesser extent excess salt in our diets play key roles in the development of hypertension.
- Eating less salt and maintaining a healthy weight can lower blood pressure, and prevent heart disease and stroke.

---

216 Coronary heart disease was reduced by 17%, stroke 27%, and all-cause mortality by 13%. The absolute risk reduction (benefit to the individual) was 1.35%, but the published paper does not specify over how many years.

32. Alcohol

It is said that microbes invented alcohol, but mammals mastered it.

The term 'alcohol' first appeared around the end of the Middle Ages. It is a derivation of the Arabic word al-khul which means body-eating spirit. The first record of beer is on Sumerian cuneiform tablets and Egyptian hieroglyphic inscriptions dating back more than 5000 years[217]. The first mention of wine is on pottery shards in Jiahu, central China[465] and pottery fragments from Georgia in the South Caucasus.[466] The Irish claim Saint Patrick was the first to distil whiskey[218,] and the oldest whiskey distillery in Ireland is Bushmills. It began production in 1608 and remains in operation today. The Scots say the monk Magnus Eunson, better known for his smuggling exploits, first illegally made whisky in the Orkney Islands in the 1790s, thirty years before being granted a licence. In the United States, in the late 1800s, the Reverend Elijah Craig created the charred barrels used to produce bourbon. I'm sorry to blow these myths away. The first mention of spirits dates back to ancient Egypt from around 3,000 BC[219].

Most of the alcohol we drink is metabolised in our livers, some is excreted in our urine, and a small amount is exhaled in the air we breathe – which is how blood alcohol can be tested with a breathalyser. Several ways alcohol could affect our risk of a heart attack or stroke have been suggested. Observational studies have claimed both a beneficial and a harmful effect of drinking alcohol on the risk of heart attack or stroke.[467–474, 474b]

A detailed 2017 analysis of 45 studies raised significant doubts about the alleged benefit of alcohol in terms of protecting us against heart attacks.[475] At one stage it was incorrectly suggested that the French penchant for alcohol may explain the French paradox discussed in a previous chapter.

As discussed in Chapter 19 (*see* p.65), association does not prove causation. Various studies have shown conflicting results. Alcohol may or may not cause or protect us from stroke and heart attack depending on how much we drink in a single sitting or over many years. However, long-term excess alcohol can cause terrible damage to our bodies, including:

- cirrhosis of the liver, leading to fluid build-up in the legs and abdomen
- swollen veins in the gullet[220,] which can rupture and cause torrential and life-threatening bleeding, and
- in men, shrinking of the testes and growth of breast tissue.

Excess alcohol can also damage our brains causing dementia and ataxia (unsteadiness). We can lose our ability to walk due to damage to the nerves

---

217 David M. Kiefer © American Chemical Society 2001:
     http://pubs.acs.org/subscribe/archive/tcaw/10/i12/html/12chemchron.html.
218 The Irish spell it whiskey, the Scots whisky.
219 The history of whisky Maison du Whisky: https://www.whisky.fr/en/history-of-whisky.
220 These are called oesophageal varices.

(peripheral neuropathy) or muscles (myopathy) in our legs. We can become very short of breath and swell up when alcohol damages our hearts (cardiomyopathy). Problems can also occur if we drink too much at one time. Alcohol levels over 0.05 lead to motor vehicle accidents. It is less well-known that intoxication increases our risk of drowning, head injuries from falls, and acute pancreatitis[221] (inflammation in the pancreas gland that sits just below the stomach on the left side of our abdomen). Pancreatitis can be fatal; drinking too much alcohol in a short space of time can also be fatal. John Bonham, the drummer for rock band Led Zeppelin and Bon Scott, the lead singer for AC/DC, had both been drinking very heavily when they died by inhaling their own vomit. Bonham had drunk 40 shots of vodka in 24 hours!

Alcohol and Blood Pressure

Studying how alcohol affects our health is challenging for several reasons. Heavy drinkers are less likely to participate in surveys, people often underestimate how much they drink, and drinking habits are hard to measure.[476] Obesity in drinkers is also rarely discussed.

Many studies have linked alcohol to high blood pressure. A 2020 review[477] looked at how alcohol affects blood pressure in the short term. It found that drinking less than 30 grams (about three standard drinks) can lower blood pressure for up to six hours, without raising it. Drinking more than 30 grams can lower blood pressure for up to 12 hours, but after that, it increases.

Long-term studies suggest that drinking alcohol daily, especially without food, may increase the risk of high blood pressure.[478,479] Some research found that people with high blood pressure also had a higher body mass index(BMI),[479] but other studies did not find this link.[478] One possible reason alcohol raises blood pressure is that it affects the inner lining, the "Teflon" of the arteries.[480]

Each standard drink (10 grams of alcohol) contains about 70 calories (290 kJ). A standard drink is 275ml of 5% beer, 100ml of white wine, 88ml of red wine, or 30ml of spirits.[481] Drinking more alcohol means consuming more calories, which can lead to weight gain and higher blood pressure.

How Much Alcohol Is Safe?

In the 19th century, Germans recommended that everyone, including children, could drink a quart (1.1L or 37oz) of beer a day[222]. Today, Australian guidelines advise no more than 10 standard drinks per week and no more than four in a single day. French guidelines are similar, while Italians allow up to 2.5 standard drinks per day. The International Alliance for Responsible Drinking provides information on alcohol recommendations for different countries[223].

---

221 I have seen an 18-year-old man die of pancreatitis. The first time he drank alcohol; he had imbibed an entire bottle of spirits!

222 New York Public Library picture collection https://www.theatlantic.com/international/archive/2012/10/germans-used-to-drink-an-astounding-amount-of-beer/263944/.

223 http://www.iard.org/policy-tables/drinking-guidelines-general-population/.

33. Smoking

Although some of us may have a relative who smoked like a chimney and died at 95, most smokers will not be so lucky.

There was a time during the 20th century when smoking was very fashionable!

Figure 33.1 An advertisement where Ronal Reagan is saying "I am giving my friends Chesterfield cigarettes for Christmas!

Smoking is one of the most important and preventable risk factors for stroke (and heart attacks).

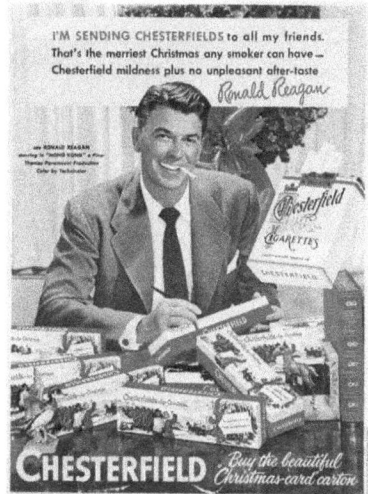

Tobacco comes from the leaves of the Nicotiana plant, which belongs to the nightshade family and is native to North and South America. Humans likely discovered tobacco around 18,000 years ago, and people began farming it between 3,000 and 5,000 BC.[482]

Archaeologists believe the Maya people in Central America were the first to use tobacco, smoking it in religious ceremonies as early as the first century BC.[483] Christopher Columbus introduced tobacco to Europe in the 15th century, but it wasn't until the 16th century that a Frenchman named Jean Nicot (after whom nicotine is named) helped make it popular.

The dangers of smoking were first suspected in the 18th century. In 1761, Dr. John Hill, a London physician, published a study linking excessive use of snuff (powdered tobacco inhaled through the nostril) with cancer of the nose. In 1795 a German doctor, Samuel Thomas von Soemmerring, noticed a connection between pipe smoking and lip cancer. Earlier in the same century Sir Francis Bacon first recognised that tobacco was addictive.[484]

In the 20th century, scientists found a clear link between smoking and lung cancer.[217,485,486] In 1964, the US Surgeon General Luther L. Terry released a report showing that smoking increased the risk of lung cancer by 10 times and also raised the risk of heart disease.[487] However, tobacco companies denied these dangers for nearly 50 years.

In 1999, US President Bill Clinton and the Department of Justice sued the tobacco industry. As a result, tobacco companies had to pay billions in compensation.

Smoking rates in the US dropped by 60% to about 13%.[488] However, in many other countries, especially in Asia, smoking is still common. Globally, about 25% of men smoke, with half of them living in China, India, or Indonesia.[489]

Smoking damages the inner lining (intima or Teflon-like layer) of our arteries and increases the risk of strokes and heart attacks. Studies show that smoking can raise this risk by up to four times.[490–503] Second-hand smoke (breathing in smoke from other people) can increase the risk of stroke by 1.5 to 2 times.[492,504,505] Although John Bailar III has expressed concern about the quality of the data and states that *"we still do not know, with accuracy, how much or even whether exposure to environmental tobacco smoke increases the risk of coronary heart disease".*[218]

Smoking even one cigarette a day can raise the risk of heart attacks and strokes,[502,506] and the risk increases the more someone smokes.[502,503,507,508] Research suggests that for every extra five cigarettes a person smokes each day, their risk of serious health problems rises by 12%.[503]

E-cigarettes, or vapes, heat liquid to create an aerosol that users inhale. This liquid may contain nicotine, THC (the chemical in marijuana that makes people feel "high"), CBD oils, and other additives. Some people use e-cigarettes to quit smoking, but it's unclear if they are safer. Vapes still contain nicotine, which harms the arteries and increases the risk of heart disease.[509]

A vaping related lung disease called EVALI (electronic-cigarette, or vaping product, use–associated lung injury) was first identified in 2019. It can cause severe breathing problems, sometimes landing people in intensive care, and has led to several deaths; vitamin E additives may be to blame.[510]

The good news is that quitting smoking improves health. The earlier someone quits, the better. Stroke risk decreases, and life expectancy improves.[488,511] After five years without smoking, heart disease risk lowers, though former heavy smokers still have a higher risk than those who never smoked.[512] Switching to cigars or pipes don't seem to help.[513]

We have already mentioned Thomas Sydenham's quote, that a man is as old as his arteries. Smoking ages the arteries by 10 years, making quitting one of the best ways to protect long-term health.[514]

How Smoking Increases our Risk

We've already talked about how important the inner lining of our arteries (called the intima), is in protecting the artery walls from damage. Several things in cigarette smoke, including carbon monoxide, nicotine, and free radicals, contribute to damage to the intima.[515,516] This leads to more serious atherosclerosis[517] (where arteries narrow due to plaque build-up). Nicotine is thought to make this problem worse.[509]

Smoking also increases the risk of stroke because it makes tiny blood cells called platelets stick together, forming small clots. These platelet clots can trigger larger blood clots that cause heart attacks and strokes. Even smoking just two cigarettes can have this effect, and aspirin does not seem to prevent it.[518]

Does Decreasing Smoking Help?

Cutting down on smoking can lower the risk of lung cancer.[519] There is conflicting evidence as to whether just cutting down how much we smoke decreases our risk of heart attacks and stroke.[520, 521]

The evidence is conflicting, other studies suggest that for light smokers, the risk of heart attack and stroke returns to normal after about five years of quitting, but for heavy smokers it can take more than 25 years. However, quitting at any time is still better than continuing to smoke. It can reduce the risk of further health problems by about one-third.

34. Sleep Apnoea

Sleep apnoea is sometimes called Pickwickian syndrome, named after a character in Charles Dickens' book *The Pickwick Papers* who had similar symptoms.

Sleep apnoea is often linked to obesity. People with this condition snore loudly and may stop breathing for more than 10 seconds at a time while sleeping. This can happen many times a night and can cause frequent waking to gasp for air. As a result, people with sleep apnoea feel extremely tired during the day and may have headaches in the morning.

The most common type is obstructive sleep apnoea (OSA), where the throat muscles collapse and block the airway. A rarer type, called central sleep apnoea, is caused by problems in the brain. Some people may have both forms.

A partner or spouse often notices sleep apnoea first. Doctors confirm the diagnosis using a sleep study, which measures how often breathing stops or slows during sleep. The severity of OSA is measured using something called the apnoea-hypopnoea index (AHI), a score based on how many times breathing slows or stops during sleep. Mild OSA is 5–14 times per hour, moderate is 15–29, and severe is 30 or more. Drinking alcohol can make sleep apnoea worse.[522,523]

In 2022, the Agency for Healthcare Research and Quality (AHRQ), an independent organisation, reported that sleep medicine has not clearly defined OSA. They found 13 different definitions of hypopnoea (abnormally slow or shallow breathing), which has led to major differences in how the AHI score is calculated.[524]

OSA is linked to an irregular heartbeat (arrhythmia, in particular atrial fibrillation[224]). While most of these irregular heartbeats are not life-threatening, some serious ones can happen, but they are not significantly more common in people with OSA.[525] Sleep apnoea also increases the risk of car accidents[526,527] and may be linked to sudden death[528–534] and stroke.[529,531,532] However, it is not clear whether OSA itself causes these problems or if other health conditions, like obesity and high blood pressure, play a bigger role.

It is still unknown whether OSA alone, without heart disease, can cause sudden death.[535] Stroke, heart attacks, and cardiac arrest are rarely seen during sleep studies[225].

A review of eight randomised trials involving a total of 5,817 participants concluded that there is no evidence that CPAP prevented heart attack or stroke.[536]

---

224 Atrial fibrillation aka AF is where the small chambers in our hearts, the atria, do not contract normally, increasing the risk of blood clot formation inside the chamber.

225 I asked three sleep study centres if they had seen stroke, heart attack or cardiac arrest during a sleep study. None had occurred in one unit during 8,000 studies over 30 years. In the other, two sleep laboratories that combined do 90 studies per week, not one case of cardiac arrest, heart attack or stroke occurred during a study.

Treatment

The most common treatment for OSA_{226} is **continuous positive airway pressure (CPAP)**,[537] which uses a machine to keep the airway open during sleep. However, only about one-third of people continue using CPAP long-term.[538] Other treatments include:

- **Oral appliances** (mouth guards or splints) that help keep the airway open.[539,540]
- **Sleeping on the stomach or side** instead of the back$_{227}$.[541]
- **Weight loss**, which is the best way to reduce OSA and other health risks. Losing about 3 kg can lower the severity of OSA by 7%.[542] More significant weight loss of 18% body weight (-21kg) lead to a 40–50% decrease in the AHI.[543]

CPAP improves sleep quality, reduces snoring, and makes people feel more awake during the day. However, studies have not proven that CPAP prevents heart attacks, strokes, or early death. The best way to improve long-term health is to maintain a healthy weight.

In 2022, the US Preventive Services Task Force concluded that there was not enough evidence for or against routine screening for OSA, and that it was not possible to assess the benefits of treating OSA in terms of cardiovascular (heart attacks) and cerebrovascular events (strokes).[544]

Conclusion

Sleep apnoea causes excessive tiredness and can affect quality of life.[545] CPAP helps people sleep better and feel more energetic, but it has not been proven to extend life[536] Losing weight is the best way to treat sleep apnoea and improve overall health.

---

226 Recommended by the American Academy of Sleep Medicine.
227 I have personally observed the benefit of sleeping on the side with a pillow behind the back in a travelling companion with whom I shared a room.

35. Irregular Heartbeat
– Atrial Fibrillation

Atrial fibrillation (AF) is a condition where the upper chambers of the heart (atria) do not beat properly. Instead of contracting normally, they quiver like a bag of wriggling worms. This can cause blood to pool and form clots, increasing the risk of stroke.

Symptoms of AF can include a fluttering feeling in the chest (palpitations), shortness of breath, dizziness if blood pressure drops, tiredness, and trouble exercising. It becomes more common as people get older.[546,547]

There are different types of AF:

- **Subclinical AF**: No symptoms, but AF is present.
- **Paroxysmal AF**: Episodes that come and go on their own.
- **Persistent AF**: Lasts more than seven days and may need treatment to stop.
- **Permanent AF**: Long-term AF that does not go away.

The Framingham study was the first to find a link between AF and stroke,[548–550] and many studies have confirmed this connection.[551–554] Blood thinners can help lower the risk of stroke for people with AF.

Strokes in people with AF tend to be more severe and sometimes fatal,[555] although they can be discovered on a CT scan[229] even in people with no stroke symptoms. The risk increases if AF episodes last longer or happen more often.[556–558] Even people with silent (sub-clinical) AF have a higher stroke risk.[559,560]

Doctors use scoring systems to estimate stroke risk, in people with AF. One of these is the CHA_2DS_2-VASc Score, which gives points based on different risk factors[228].

Our risk of stroke is greater with an increased score, as shown in Table 35.1.

CHA_2DS_2-VASc Score	% risk of stroke per year[561]	
	Males	Females
0	0.2	The minimum score is 1*
1	0.6	0.6
2	2.2	2.2
3	3.2	3.2
4	4.8	4.8
5	7.2	7.2
6	9.7	9.7
7	11.2	11.2
8	10.6	10.8
9	Maximum Score 8*	12.2

Table 35.1. The CHA_2DS_2-VASc score used to estimate the risk of stroke in patients with atrial fibrillation. Why the risk with a score of 8 is less than with 7 is uncertain. * Being female scores 1 as opposed to male who scores zero, thus the minimum score for a female is 1 and the maximum score for a male is 8. Professor Gregory Lip from the faculty of Health and Life Sciences, University of Liverpool, UK, created the CHA_2DS_2-VASc score.

228 https://www.mdcalc.com/calc/801/cha2ds2-vasc-score-atrial-fibrillation-stroke-risk#:~:text=The%20CHA2DS2,patient's%20risk%20for%20TE%20event.

If someone has a CHA$_2$DS$_2$-VASc score of 2 or more, they are usually advised to take blood thinners (anticoagulants) to help prevent strokes (see Chapter 43[229]).

Even though having atrial fibrillation (AF) increases stroke risk, AF is not always the direct cause of a stroke. Doctors need to check for other possible causes in every stroke patient. **People under 65 years old with lone AF** (meaning they have none of the risk factors in Table 35.1) **have a very low stroke risk – about 0.6% per year for women and 0.2% for men.**

Some studies suggest that AF might not cause strokes; that there must be another cause. This is because research looking at recordings from heart monitors (loop recorders) implanted in some patients found that very few had AF in the month leading up to and at the time of their stroke.[562] Another reason is that a test called a transoesophageal echocardiogram (TOE[230]), which can check for blood clots in the heart, only finds them in about 10% of patients with AF.[563] If someone with AF takes warfarin (a blood thinner) for at least four weeks, their risk of having a visible clot drops to 1.9%, and it is zero in those with lone AF.[564]

Long-term (chronic or permanent) AF enlarges the heart's atria (upper chambers),[565] and some experts believe this may be why AF is linked to strokes – not the irregular heartbeat itself. The Framingham study found that a larger left atrium increased stroke risk in men and death risk in both men and women.[566] An enlarged left atrium leads to blood clot formation in the absence of AF.

Contrarian Thought
People with lone AF have a very low risk of stroke. The factors used in the CHA$_2$DS$_2$-VASc score to assess stroke risk – such as older age, high blood pressure, diabetes, past strokes, and vascular disease – are the same factors that increase the risk of stroke in people without AF. Since blood clots cause strokes, it makes sense that the blood thinners used to treat AF should also help prevent strokes caused by blood clots in people without AF. However, studies have not been able to clearly show that warfarin works better than aspirin for preventing strokes in people who do not have AF.[567–569]
It would be interesting to see if blood thinners would be helpful in patients without AF who have a CHA$_2$DS$_2$-Vasc score of 3 or more.

---

229 Chapters 41–47 and the references can be found at www.understandingneurology.com.au.
230 TEE or transesophageal echocardiography in the US.

36. Physical Activity

To bring a personal perspective, the author is a keen cyclist[231] and golfer who exercises regularly to stay fit and maintain his health – and therefore may be a little biased in his views on exercise.

So far, the discussion has focused on risk factors that **increase** the risk of heart disease and stroke, but many believe that exercise can help **lower** this risk. Unfortunately, most people do not get enough exercise to stay healthy. The World Health Organization (WHO) warns that lack of physical activity will lead to nearly 500 million cases of heart disease, obesity, diabetes, and other serious health problems between 2020 and 2030. The cost of treating these preventable diseases is expected to reach almost $300 billion by 2030[232].

Exercise is clearly beneficial when it leads to weight loss, as this can lower blood pressure, cholesterol, and diabetes risk. However, even without weight loss,[570,571] exercise may still help reduce heart disease risk in other ways. Aerobic exercise can make arteries more flexible, lower blood pressure,[572,573] and slow the resting heart rate,[574] which is linked to a lower risk of heart attack, stroke, and early death. An elevated resting heart rate increases our risk of heart attack,[575] stroke,[576] and death from all causes.[577]

Contrarian Thought
The fitter we are, the lower our resting heartbeat: the benefits of exercise may come from having a slower heart rate, which reduces stress on the arteries simply because blood is pumped into our arteries less often.

Some studies suggest that regular exercise can improve how the body processes glucose in people with diabetes,[578,579] though its impact on heart disease risk is uncertain.[580–584] Research on exercise and cholesterol levels has produced mixed results.[585–587] In some cases, exercise slightly increases "good" HDL cholesterol, but it does not significantly lower "bad" LDL cholesterol unless paired with weight loss.[588]

Animal studies have also shown conflicting results. In some cases, exercise improved cholesterol levels and reduced artery disease[233],[589] but in others, it did not.[590]

Two long forgotten studies of Harvard graduates[591] and longshoremen[234],[592] suggested that those who exercised[235] more had lower death rates, but these

---

231 I ride 120–150km per week.
232 https://www.who.int/news/item/19-10-2022-who-highlights-high-cost-of-physical-inactivity-in-first-ever-global-report.
233 At autopsy, there was less atherosclerosis in the arteries of the monkeys that exercised.
234 Waterside or dock workers.
235 Death rates were one-quarter to one-third lower in the Harvard group who were expending an excess of 2,000 Calories per week with exercise and halved in the longshoreman who expended the most energy (an excess of 1876 Calories/day), as opposed to their more sedentary (half as many Calories) work colleagues. Calories (with a capital C) refers to kilocalories. There are 4.2 Calories per kJ. The recommended consumption of Calories is 2,000–2,500 per day.

studies did not consider other factors like weight, smoking, or high blood pressure. More recent research based on UK Biobank data[593–595] suggests that moderate to vigorous exercise[236] lowers the risk of heart disease, and even short bursts of intense activity provide benefits.

An Expression of Concern
Studies on exercise and heart disease are observational, meaning they show a link but do not prove cause and effect. They also do not account for weight loss, which could be the real reason for the health benefits seen in people who exercise more. It is hard to believe that those, such as the longshoreman, burning in excess of 1,000 more calories per day remained overweight or were not thinner than those undertaking little exercise.

Guidelines published in 2018[596,597] recommend at least 150–300 minutes of exercise per week[237]. Exercise has benefits beyond heart health, including reducing the risk of cancer, improving brain function, boosting mental health, and preventing falls in older adults.[598] Strength training is especially helpful for maintaining muscle strength and mobility in older people.

We are never too old to exercise. However, while exercise has many benefits, it also carries some risks. Intense activity, such as cycling, gym and running can briefly increase the chance of sudden cardiac death,[599,600] but this risk is very low – about one case per million hours of exercise.[601] The Framingham study showed that the life-time risk of sudden death for a 45-year-old is 10.9% in men and 2.8% in women.[602] For young people, sudden death is usually caused by genetic heart conditions, while in older adults, it is often due to underlying heart disease. If someone decides to start exercising later in life, it is wise to get a health check first and gradually increase intensity under expert guidance to avoid injury.

A famous example is Jim Fixx, author of *The Complete Book of Running*, who died of a heart attack at age 52 while running. He had started exercising later in life after years of smoking and being overweight, showing that past lifestyle choices can still impact future health.

Summary

Exercise has the most benefit for our hearts and blood vessels when it leads to weight loss and is done regularly at higher intensities. If someone is returning to exercise in mid-life, they should start slowly, under supervision, and seek medical advice to reduce risks.

---

236 The risk of ASCVD was 14% lower with exercise that burnt 15KJ (3.6 calories)/kg/day and 39% lower with exercise that burnt 60KJ (14.3 calories)/kg/day. The benefit increased to a 47% risk reduction when 60% of the 60KJ/kg/day was burnt doing moderate-vigorous exercise. If I have interpreted this study correctly, an 80 kg individual would achieve the maximum benefit by exercising at a moderate-vigorous intensity burning an extra 4,800 KJ (1,142 calories) daily. That is a great deal of exercise; if they did not increase their intake of calories, they would have lost weight. Was it just the exercise, or was it the weight loss that led to the benefit?

237 This would be 20–45 minutes daily.

SECTION 10:
Heart Attacks

Although this book primarily focuses on the causes and prevention of stroke, much of its content is even more relevant to **ischaemic heart disease (IHD)**, causing heart attacks and angina.

Ischaemic heart disease is a condition where the heart does not get enough oxygen-rich blood because the arteries are blocked or narrowed. It is also known as coronary heart disease or coronary artery disease.

Angina is a temporary chest pain caused by reduced blood flow in the arteries that supply blood to the heart. It does not cause permanent damage. Angina is often triggered by physical exertion and relieved by rest. Like heart attack pain, it can also radiate to the jaw and left arm.

Atherosclerosis is the primary cause of IHD, and much of what is discussed in this book applies to it as well. For this reason, I have included a brief chapter on IHD.

37. Angina and Heart Attacks

Atherosclerosis is the underlying disease causing 90% of heart attacks. In the other 10% of patients who suffer a heart attack, the coronary arteries (arteries to the heart) look normal on angiography (an imaging procedure used to check blood vessels).[603–605] Some of these heart attacks are thought to be related to mild atheroma that modern tests cannot detect, and some are due to spasm of our coronary artery. There are other extremely rare causes that are beyond the scope of this book.

Heart attacks occur in patients under the age of 30 where the only risk factors are smoking[606,607] or obesity. Obesity is the only risk factor in 30% of patients under the age of 40 who have heart attacks.[606,607]

Atherosclerosis (plaque or coronary artery calcification) that does not cause any symptoms can happen in people without any of the traditional risk factors. 17.6% of 136,905 patients admitted with coronary artery disease had LDL cholesterol levels < 70 mg/dL (1.81 mmol/L).[114] Twenty-seven percent of patients admitted to hospital with a heart attack do not have any of the so-called risk factors.[113]

Alarmingly the incidence of heart attacks, angina and sudden death, i.e. ischaemic heart disease (IHD), is increasing in 15–30-year-olds. In 2019 globally it had reached 26.81 (95% uncertainty interval [UI]: 20.36−34.54) per 100,000.[608]

As atherosclerosis becomes more severe, tiny specks of calcium build up in the walls of our arteries. This build up typically occurs after the age of 40 (decades after atherosclerosis commences), and most people older than age 60 will have scattered calcification.[609,610] The amount of calcium in our coronary arteries can be measured by an electron beam CT scan.[611] This is called the Coronary Artery Calcium Score (CAC).

The higher the CAC score, the more likely we are to have more severe atherosclerosis. If the score is 0, the likelihood of **mild plaques of atheroma** is 7.4% and the likelihood of a **narrow coronary artery** is 5.8%. On the other hand, if the score is 200 or more the likelihood is 39.7 and 60.3% respectively.[612]

The 10 and 15 year-risk of **stroke or heart attack** with a CAC score of 0 is only 1–3% respectively. If the CAC score is more than 400, this risk increases to 20–28%.[613,614]

An increased CAC score occurs in about one-third of us deemed to have a low 10-year risk (<7.5%) using the ASCVD risk score, and can identify those of us who have a threefold (4.33 vs 1.41 per thousand patient years) increased risk of developing symptoms of ASCVD.[615] The things we can do to reduce our risk of heart attack are the same things that will reduce our risk of stroke. Namely, not smoke and avoid obesity. If we have obesity, then weight loss can eliminate high blood pressure, high cholesterol and diabetes,[616] and greatly reduce our risk – as was seen in West Germany and Finland at the end and shortly after World War II. The next two chapters deal with weight control.

The severity of coronary artery calcification (the CAC score) increases with age, particularly over 65 and more so in men than women. Coronary artery calcification is detected in 40% and 22% of men and women respectively under the age of 45. At 75 or older this increases to 86% in men and 80% in women. The median calcium score is > 400 in men and > 100 in women 75 years and older. The CAC score is unrelated to the total and the LDL cholesterol levels. For men, median calcium scores were not significantly different for the LDL-C or the total cholesterol levels while women displayed either minimal or no calcified plaque for these variables.[616a]

In symptomatic patients with severely elevated LDL-C levels of at least 190 mg/dL (4.9 mmol/L) who are universally considered to be at high risk by guidelines, the absence of calcified and non-calcified plaque on coronary computed tomographic angiography was associated with low risk for ASCVD events.[612]

The CAC score is a better predictor of the severity of the underlying coronary atherosclerosis and subsequent ASCVD (heart attack, stroke and death) than LDL levels. In adjusted analyses, absence vs presence of CAC was associated with markedly lower risk for events in all LDL-C groups.[612]

SECTION 11:
Calories, Exercise and Weight Loss

The massive rise in obesity, along with its complications of high blood pressure, high cholesterol, and diabetes, has fuelled an epidemic of heart attacks, strokes, and poor circulation in the legs.

In the 1950s, the obesity rate was **5.8%**. By 1990, it had increased to 14.8%[238] [617] and is projected to reach **49% by 2030**.[618] Alarmingly, childhood and adolescent obesity rates are also rising. Between 1970 and 1990, obesity prevalence among urban African American adolescents tripled in males and quadrupled in females.[619]

A **2022 WHO report**[239] stated that **one in eight people worldwide** were living with obesity:

- Adult obesity worldwide has **more than doubled** since 1990, while adolescent obesity has **quadrupled.**
- In 2022, **2.5 billion** adults aged 18 and older (43.5%) were overweight, including **890 million** (16%) living with obesity.
- In 2022, **37 million children under the age of five** were overweight.
- Over **390 million children and adolescents (aged 5–19 years)** were overweight in 2022, including **160 million** living with obesity.

This surge in obesity is mainly because people are eating too many calories – particularly from **highly processed, addictive, and appetite-stimulating carbohydrates** – and are also increasingly less active.

As seen during the later years of and soon after **World War II**, as well as following **bariatric surgery**, weight loss can **reduce and potentially eliminate** the risk of obesity-related diseases.

The next two chapters explore **calories, exercise, medications, and surgical options** for weight loss.

---

238 This comes from the Framingham Study.
239 https://www.who.int/news-room/fact-sheets/detail/obesity-and-overweight.

38. Calories in Calories out

Losing weight can reduce the severity of atherosclerosis, losing massive amounts of weight can reverse atherosclerosis. Our weight depends on the balance between how many calories we eat and how many we burn. It's that simple. The problem is that in today's world, it's hard to control how much we eat. Many people try crash diets, but often regain any lost weight when they go back to old eating habits. To truly lower the risk of heart attacks and strokes, we need to commit to lifelong healthy eating to prevent weight gain or keep off any weight we lose.

This chapter explains how many calories our bodies need, how different activities burn calories, and how much exercise it takes to burn off common foods like a hamburger, a packet of chips, a soft drink, or ice cream.

Table 38.1 lists our daily calorie needs according to age, sex, and level of physical activity. On average, people who are very active burn **400–600 more calories per day** than those who are inactive. As we get older, our bodies need fewer calories. By the time we reach our 80s, we need **400–600 fewer calories** per day than we did in our 20s.

Table 38.2 lists how many calories we "burn" with various types of exercise. Different exercises burn different amounts of calories, and some foods take a surprising amount of effort to work off.

Table 38.3 shows how much exercise we need to do to burn off the calories in popular food and beverages. For example, if we just sit and watch TV, it would take **10–12 hours** to burn off the calories from a single hamburger. This makes it clear why losing weight can be so difficult.

Estimated Calorie Needs per Day

	Males				Females		
AGE	Sedentary [a]	Moderately Active [b]	Active [c]	AGE	Sedentary [a]	Moderately Active [b]	Active [c]
2	1,000	1,000	1,000	2	1,000	1,000	1,000
3	1,000	1,400	1,400	3	1,000	1,400	1,400
4	1,200	1,400	1,600	4	1,200	1,400	1,600
5	1,200	1,400	1,600	5	1,200	1,400	1,600
6	1,400	1,600	1,800	6	1,400	1,600	1,800
7	1,400	1,600	1,800	7	1,400	1,600	1,800
8	1,400	1,600	2,000	8	1,400	1,600	2,000
9	1,600	1,800	2,000	9	1,600	1,800	2,000
10	1,600	1,800	2,200	10	1,600	1,800	2,200
11	1,800	2,000	2,200	11	1,800	2,000	2,200
12	1,800	2,200	2,400	12	1,800	2,200	2,400
13	2,000	2,200	2,600	13	2,000	2,200	2,600

Males				Females			
AGE	Sedentary [a]	Moderately Active [b]	Active [c]	AGE	Sedentary [a]	Moderately Active [b]	Active [c]
14	2,000	2,400	2,800	14	2,000	2,400	2,800
15	2,200	2,600	3,000	15	2,200	2,600	3,000
16	2,400	2,800	3,200	16	2,400	2,800	3,200
17	2,400	2,800	3,200	17	2,400	2,800	3,200
18	2,400	2,800	3,200	18	2,400	2,800	3,200
19–20	2,600	2,800	3,000	19–20	2,600	2,800	3,000
21–25	2,400	2,800	3,000	21–25	2,400	2,800	3,000
26–30	2,400	2,600	3,000	26–30	2,400	2,600	3,000
31–35	2,400	2,600	3,000	31–35	2,400	2,600	3,000
36–40	2,400	2,600	2,800	36–40	2,400	2,600	2,800
41–45	2,200	2,600	2,800	41–45	2,200	2,600	2,800
46–50	2,200	2,400	2,800	46–50	2,200	2,400	2,800
51–55	2,200	2,400	2,800	51–55	2,200	2,400	2,800
56–60	2,200	2,400	2,600	56–60	2,200	2,400	2,600
61–65	2,000	2,400	2,600	61–65	2,000	2,400	2,600
66–70	2,000	2,200	2,600	66–70	2,000	2,200	2,600
71–75	2,000	2,200	2,600	71–75	2,000	2,200	2,600
≥ 76	2,000	2,200	2,400	≥ 76	2,000	2,200	2,400

Table 38.1. Age vs Daily Energy in Calories for age, sex, and level of physical activity
[a] Sedentary means only doing basic daily activities, like moving around the house.
[b] Moderately active means doing some extra movement, like walking 2.4–4.8 km per day at a moderate pace, along with basic daily activities.
[c] Active means doing even more exercise, like walking more than 4.8 km per day at a moderate pace, along with basic daily activities.
[d] These calorie estimates do not include extra needs for pregnant or breastfeeding women.

Source: Institute of Medicine. Dietary Reference Intakes for Energy, Carbohydrate, Fiber, Fat, Fatty Acids, Cholesterol, Protein, and Amino Acids. Washington (DC): The National Academies Press; 2002. https://health.gov/sites/default/files/2019-09/2015-2020_Dietary_Guidelines.pdf.

Exercise and Calorie Consumption

Activity	MET* Value	Calories per hour
Sleeping	1.0	93
Sitting	1.5	140
Walking slowly	3.8	355
Walking briskly	4.5	420
Jogging	7.0	654
Running fast 14 km/h (8.7 mph)	12.3	1140
Elite marathon runner ** 20 km/h (12 mph)	19	1064
Recreational swimming	5.8	542
Vigorous swimming	9.8	916

Activity	MET* Value	Calories per hour
Exercise class	5.5	514
Cycling slowly 9km/h (5.6 mph)	3.5	327
Cycling vigorously 24km/h (15 mph)	14	1308

Table 38.2. *Calories burned during different activities or exercises can be measured using METs, which stands for Metabolic Equivalent. MET is a way to show how hard an exercise is.[620,621] The numbers in the table show the average for different types of exercise. The right column shows the calorie burn for an average male weighing 89kg[240]. To calculate how many calories are burned in a minute, use this formula: MET score x 3.5 x body weight (in kg) ÷ 200. To get the number of calories burned in an hour, multiply the result by 60. **Note The average weight for a male marathon runner is 56.2kg.

Table 38.3 shows why it is so hard to burn all the calories from highly processed, calorie-dense foods and drinks.

Time to Burn Calories from Food

	599–1381 Kcal * (2508–5778Kj)	1 Bag ** 2112Kj (505 Kcal)	160–538 Kcal *** (669–2251Kj)	274 Kcal **** 1146Kj
Sitting (140)	4.3–9.9	3.6–7.2	1.1–3.8	1.95
Gentle Cycling (327)	1.8–4.2	1.5–3.1	29–1.6	50
Walking Briskly (420)	1.42–3.3	1.2–2.4	23–1.3	39
Jogging (654)	55–2.1	46–1.5	15–49	25
Swimming (916)	39–1.5	33–1.1	11–35	17
Running (1140)	32–1.2	27–53	8–28	14
Cycling hard (1308)	27–1.1	23–46	7–25	13

Table 38.3. The amount of exercise needed to burn off the calories in different foods (shown in brackets as calories per hour). *Depends on the type of hamburger. **The packet size ranges from 227–380 grams (13.4oz). ***The drink sizes range from 330ml to 1.25L (11.2–43.3 oz). **** 2 scoops. The grey numbers show minutes, while the black numbers show hours. The first line of numbers below the pictures shows how many calories are in the food. The calorie content in the food and beverages can be found at the FOOD Standards Australia New Zealand website,[241] or one of the popular on-line websites such as KalorieKing[242].

240 89 kg is the average US male weight.
241 https://afcd.foodstandards.gov.au/?_gl=1*1cmq89p*_ga*ODE2Mjg4MTQuMTc0NTkyOTMzMQ..*_ga_74D9VJQ21L*MTc0NjAxNzk4OS4yLjEuMTc0NjAxNjAxODAwMy40Ni4wLjA.*_ga_97GJ8R086T*MTc0NjAxNzk4OS4yLjEuMTc0NjAxNjAxODAwMy40Ni4wLjA. (241).
242 https://www.calorieking.com/us/en/.

39. Drugs and Surgery for Weight Loss

Drug-Induced Weight Loss

Finding a drug that safely causes significant weight loss is the goal of many scientists. In 2018, researchers managed to block a gene called RCAN1 in mice, allowing them to eat as much fatty food as they wanted without gaining weight. Instead of storing fat, the mice turned it into energy.[622,623] It will take years to find out if this can work in humans and if it's safe.

Drugs like ephedrine and caffeine, which are in some foods and supplements, can help with a small amount of weight loss.

There have been several drugs developed to treat obesity, but many have been withdrawn because of side effects[243].[624–626]

The US Food and Drug Administration (FDA) has approved some drugs for weight loss, such as **orlistat**[244] (Xenical, Alli), **lorcaserin** (Belviq), **phentermine-topiramate** (Qsymia) and **naltrexone-bupropion** (Contrave), but they only help people achieve 5–10% weight loss.[627–632] For example, if someone weighs 100kg, they may only lose about 5–10kg; they will still be obese.

A newer group of drugs used for weight loss, called GLP-1 receptor agonists[245], were originally developed to treat diabetes. Most GLP-1 receptor agonists are given by injection, although in 2020 an oral form was developed.[633] They help with weight loss and therefore can help prevent type 2 diabetes. They work by making people feel full, reducing binge-eating,[634,635] and decreasing hunger.[634,635] These drugs have been found to be very effective,[636–643] particularly with higher doses.[644,645] Most people lose 5–15% of their weight, not surprisingly, drug-sponsored studies[638–643] suggest some people may lose more than 10–20% of their body weight with these GLP-1 drugs, including teenagers.[646,647] There is one study, not funded by industry, that also reported a 10–20% weight loss.[648] Studies have shown that people who do not have diabetes tend to lose more weight. These drugs are usually recommended alongside exercise and a healthy diet.

They have become so popular for weight loss[649] that people with diabetes have had difficulty getting the drugs[246]. They are expensive[247] and can cause side

---

243 Fenfluramine and dexfenfluramine were withdrawn because they caused damage to heart valves. Sibutramine increased heart rate and blood pressure, caused an irregular heartbeat, and even more heart attacks. Rimonabant caused depression, anxiety, suicidal behaviour, seizures, and nausea. On February 13, 2020, the FDA asked drug company Eisai to voluntarily withdraw Belviq, their brand of appetite-suppressing drug lorcaserin, from the market because of an increased risk of pancreatic, colorectal and lung cancers.

244 Most drugs have the same generic name and a different name that individual pharmaceutical companies call their brand. The brand names are in the brackets.

245 The current GLP-1 receptor agonists include semaglutide (Ozempic, Rybelsus Wegovy), liraglutide (Saxenda), lixisenatide (Adlyxin), exenatide (Byetta), exenatide extended release (Bydureon BCise), and dulaglutide (Trulicity).

246 The current GLP-1 receptor agonists include semaglutide (Ozempic, Rybelsus Wegovy), liraglutide (Saxenda), lixisenatide (Adlyxin), exenatide (Byetta), exenatide extended release (Bydureon BCise), and dulaglutide (Trulicity).

247 More than US$4,000 per year in some cases.

effects like nausea and vomiting, inflammation of the gall bladder (cholecystitis), gall-stones and inflammation of the pancreas (pancreatitis).[650,651] Concern has been raised about the possibility of depression and suicide, although there is some doubt about these claims.[649] The delay in stomach emptying has prompted the American Society of Anesthesiologists to recommend that patients do not take GLP-1 receptor agonists on the day of surgery and stop taking their weekly dose of drugs like Wegovy seven days before a procedure[248].

However, drugs alone are not a long-term solution, as people often regain the weight once they stop taking them.[643,652,653]

An experimental drug, retatrutide, is a once-weekly drug that works in three different ways, targeting GIP (glucose-dependent insulinotropic polypeptide)[249], GLP-1[250], and glucagon receptors[251]. In early studies[654] it has been shown to reduce body weight by 3.19% to 16.94% depending on the dose.

Other Weight Loss Drugs

Other drugs are being researched for weight loss, but they are not yet approved. One of these is **topiramate**, which is used for migraines and epilepsy. While it can cause weight loss, it also has many side effects like confusion and depression, which make it hard to tolerate.[655]

Leptin, a hormone that helps regulate weight, has been tested as a weight loss treatment with claims it is effective,[656] but concerns about its safety have been raised.[657,658]

CLA[252], a substance found in meat and dairy from cows, goats, and deer, has been marketed as a fat-burning supplement. Although animal studies suggest CLA may be effective for weight loss,[659,660] the evidence for its effectiveness in human studies is weak.[661]

Surgery for Weight Loss

Surgical options are also available for treating obesity. **Liposuction** removes fat from areas like the abdomen, but it does not address deep fat inside the body, which can still cause health problems. Other methods like **CoolSculpting** and **truSculpt** use cold or heat to destroy fat cells, but these are mostly cosmetic and don't offer long-term weight loss. They may in fact be counter-productive because they cause an increase in the fat inside the abdomen (visceral fat).[662]

---

248 The reason is the risk of vomiting during surgery and aspirating the stomach contents into the lungs https://www.asahq.org/about-asa/newsroom/news-releases/2023/06/american-society-of-anesthesiologists-consensus-based-guidance-on-preoperative.

249 GIP seems to enhance the release of insulin and glucagon, and may be responsible for some cases of hypoglycemia (low blood sugar).

250 The glucagon-like peptide-1 receptor (GLP-1R) plays a crucial role in regulating blood sugar levels, lipid metabolism, and other biological functions by interacting with the hormone GLP-1.

251 Glucagon receptors, mainly found in liver cells, are crucial for maintaining glucose balance. They bind to glucagon, triggering the liver to release stored glucose (glycogen) into the bloodstream and promoting glucose production (gluconeogenesis).

252 Conjugated linoleic acid.

For people with severe obesity (BMI over 40), also called morbid obesity, weight loss surgery to the stomach called bariatric surgery may be recommended. Procedures like **gastric sleeve**, **gastric bypass**, **gastric balloon,** and **lap or gastric banding** reduce the amount of food the stomach can hold or make it harder for the body to absorb fat. These procedures are generally effective for long-term weight loss, but they come with risks like nutritional deficiencies[253] and digestive problems.[663]

Along with weight loss, bariatric surgery can help to lower blood sugar, LDL cholesterol, HbA1c levels, and blood pressure.[664] Many people who have bariatric surgery can reduce or even stop taking certain medications.[665–668] Most people, including some children, experience long-term weight loss and a better quality of life after the procedure, but not everyone.

A study of 200,000 patients with severe obesity in the US found that bariatric surgery can increase life expectancy by up to 6.7 years.[669] However, for people with extreme obesity (BMI over 62 kg/m²), the surgery might actually shorten life expectancy.

Other Procedures

AspireAssist is a method where a tube is placed through the stomach wall to remove food before the body absorbs it. It's a bit like bulimia, where people make themselves vomit after eating to avoid weight gain. But with AspireAssist, we can still enjoy eating without the discomfort of vomiting.

There are other experimental procedures, such as **bariatric embolisation** and **vagal nerve stimulation**, that aim to reduce appetite and promote weight loss. Bariatric embolisation blocks certain blood vessels to the stomach, leading to reduced appetite and some weight loss.[670] Vagal nerve stimulation uses electrical signals to decrease hunger. The idea came from the observation that people lost more weight after bariatric surgery when the vagus nerve[254] was cut.[671] Deep brain stimulation (DBS) is a well-known treatment for conditions like essential tremor and Parkinson's disease. Some researchers have tried using DBS to treat obesity. Although rats lost 40% of their weight[672,673], it is not yet a proven treatment in humans.[674] These procedures are still in the early stages of development and more research is needed to confirm their safety and effectiveness.[675]

Intragastric Botox is another experimental treatment where Botox is injected into the stomach to reduce hunger. It has shown some promise in animals,[676] but there is not enough evidence to show it works in humans.[677] As of 2022 a review found that only 192 people in total had been studied in randomised controlled trials – too few to show a benefit.[678]

---

253 Deficiencies of vitamin B12, iron, calcium, vitamin D, thiamine, folate, and the fat-soluble vitamin can occur.
254 The vagus nerve is the main nerve that sends electrical impulses from our brain to our voice box, heart, lungs, gullet (oesophagus) and our small and large bowel to control our digestion, heart rate and immune system.

Overall, while there are many options for weight loss, including drugs and surgeries, none offer a perfect or permanent solution. Lifestyle changes like exercise and healthy eating are still the most effective, but for many, a very difficult, if not impossible way to lose weight and keep it off.

40. Future Research – A Plea

Healthcare workers always want to provide the best treatment for their patients. To do this, they need clear, reliable research that can help them discuss treatment options with patients. However, some parts of the research and publishing process are causing problems. A well-known critic of this system is John Ioannidis from Stanford University, California[255].[366,679–689]

This book highlights how research funded by companies, like those in the food, medicine, and medical device industries, often shows overly positive results for the industry. This doesn't mean all industry-funded research is flawed, but it's hard to tell which studies have been influenced by industry funding. This makes it difficult to trust the research when choosing the best treatments. The British Medical Journal stopped publishing tobacco industry funded research in 2013. In 2014, they published a debate[690] titled "should journals stop publishing research funded by the drug industry?", arguing this type of research is corrupted and that companies publish it to advance their commercial aims – oblivious of the harm they do. Many recommendations were made to improve the reliability of industry-funded research. The concept of Restoring Invisible and Abandoned Trials[691] (RIAT) has been suggested as a way to encourage publication of trials that were previously misreported or which went unreported. The call[691,692] to publish invisible abandoned trials has gone unheeded. As long ago as 2004 the New York Times editors opined[256] that data sharing between pharmaceutical companies and investigators should become standard industry practice. Title VIII of the Food and Drug Administration (FDA) Amendments Act of 2007 (FDAAA) mandates that certain clinical trials involving drugs and medical devices are registered and a summary of results reported to ClinicalTrials.gov.

Sadly, however, little has changed: even with mandatory reporting, many trials are not reported on time or are reported late and as many as 60–90% are not reported at all.[257].[693–695]

---

255 Ioannidis has his critics, particularly over his raising of concerns about the reliability of data on Covid-related mortality. https://www.scientificamerican.com/article/the-ioannidis-affair-a-tale-of-major-scientific-overreaction/ This is not surprising, anyone who questions dogma is demonised, but fortunately in this modern era not executed – as they were in the Middle Ages. His PloS Medicine paper (reference 3 in the bibliography) on "Why most published research findings are false" is the most-accessed article in the history of Public Library of Science (>3 million hits).

256 https://www.nytimes.com/2004/06/06/opinion/when-drug-companies-hide-data.html.

257 A copy of the book will be sent to the National Institute of Neurological Disorders and Stroke (NINDS) with a letter expressing concern about the current method of funding and conduct of industry-sponsored research.

To improve this, the way industry funds research has to change.
- Industry continues to fund the research and choose the research sites.
- Two independent groups, funded but not chosen by the industry, should monitor the safety and data (the results of the study).
- The data should no longer be kept secret by the industry; instead, it should be held by an independent regulatory authority for public scrutiny if needed.

The Publishing Process

In terms of publishing research:
- There should be clear statements, such as "this study was or was not funded by industry" at the start of the paper$_{258}$. This would help readers quickly know if the research was industry-funded.
- Studies should also provide important information like the relative and absolute risk reduction, the numbers needed to treat, and an economic analysis of the treatment cost. This would help doctors make informed decisions with their patients. As long ago as 2010, an editorial in the highly regarded British Medical Journal made this very point. It went so far as to suggest that talking about relative risks$_{259}$ without baseline (absolute) risk is the first "sin" against transparent reporting.[696]
- A more controversial idea is whether new treatments should be tested against a placebo (a sugar pill or sham treatment) or compared with the current standard treatment. If we already have a treatment that works better than a placebo, in the opinion of this author, the new treatment should be tested against the proven treatment.

---

258 This would be less of an issue if the recommended changes in the research process listed above were adopted.
259 As discussed in Chapter 20 the relative risk is the benefit or harm to the overall population, whilst the absolute risk is the benefit or harm to the individual.

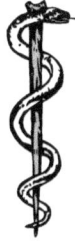

The rod of Asclepius the true symbol of medicine.

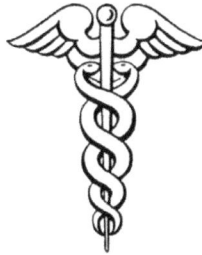

Rod of Cadaceus (the messenger of the Greek God Hermes and the Roman God Mercury) in ancient time associated with liars, thieves, trade, eloquence, negotiation, alchemy and wisdom.

The Rod of Cadaceus was incorrectly adopted by the Royal Air Force and the United States Medical Corps, Navy Pharmacy Division, and the Public Health Service in error believing it to be the symbol of medicine.

The cause of this error has its origins in the 15th century.[697,698]

The prevention and treatment of stroke is constantly changing; thus, I have elected not to put these in the published book.

The relevant chapters, the appendices that contain more complex scientific information and the references to all chapters are located at: https://www.understandingneurology.com.au/books/struck-down-by-the-gods

As we put the finishing touches to this book, there is already additional information we would like to have added. This can be found on the website:

https://www.understandingneurology.com.au/books/struck-down-by-the-gods

Not smoking and avoiding weight gain are the two things we can do as individuals to reduce our risk of stroke (and heart attack) at a younger age.

The rest is largely, but not entirely in the "Lap of the Gods". Once we develop high blood pressure, high cholesterol and diabetes treatment will also reduce our risk.

Index

G

W

X

Files on the Internet

Over the many years of researching and writing this book there have been many scientific studies that have altered how medicine prevents and treats stroke. Thus, the files dealing with treatment have been placed on a website so that they can be kept up to date. As more information becomes available after publication of this book, it will be added to the individual numbered chapters on the website

Also on the website are the appendices that discuss in greater scientific detail some of the topics in this book.

Finally on the website are links to stroke organisations where up to date information and guidelines can be found.

https://www.understandingneurology.com.au/books/struck-down-by-the-gods

Chapters

Appendices

References

https://www.understandingneurology.com.au/books/struck-down-by-the-gods

About the Author

Peter Gates

Born in Melbourne, Australia, on 7 November 1951. The eldest of six children.

Married Rosie 1979, 3 Children, Bernard, Amelia and Jeremy.

Education: Beverly Hills State School, Ivanhoe Grammar.

Graduated MB BS third class honours 1975.

Commenced Neurology Training 1980.

Admitted to Fellowship of the Royal Australian College of Physicians 1983.

Appointed Fellow of the American Academy of Neurology 2019.

The first neurologist to live and work outside the capital city of Melbourne in the state of Victoria, Australia,1986.

Established the first public hospital neurology unit in Victoria outside the capital city of Melbourne.

International teaching in Rwanda, Fiji and Sri Lanka.

Recipient of the most effective and innovative teaching award 1986.

Published highly acclaimed neurology textbook, *Clinical Neurology a primer* 2010, 2nd edition *Clinical Neurology a Cure for neurophobia* 2023

Educational website www.understandingneurology.com.au

Two-time recipient of the Richard Hallowes Prize for excellence in teaching 2005, 2006.

Awarded OAM 2021

Other interests: Keen cyclist, mediocre, but keen golfer, photography and travel.

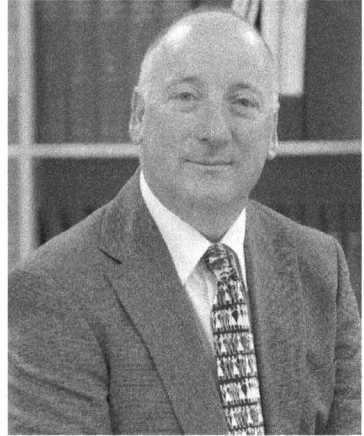

www.ingramcontent.com/pod-product-compliance
Lightning Source LLC
Chambersburg PA
CBHW041256040426
42334CB00028BA/3044